Fitness Game Plan – 2020

A Collection of Thirty-Five Ways In Seven Reports to Get You Fitter in the New Year

Ron Kness

Fitness Game Plan - 2020

No part of this book may be reproduced, stored in a retrieval system, or transmitted in any form or by any means, electronic, mechanical, photocopying, recording, scanning, or otherwise, without the prior written permission of the publisher, except for the inclusion of brief quotations in a review.

This book is for **personal use only**.

Published by:

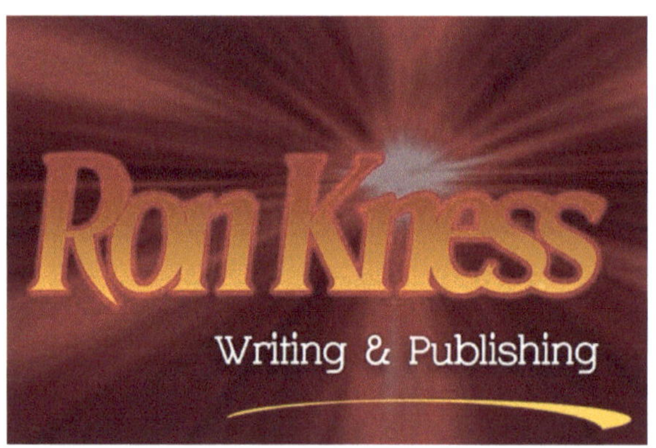

https://ronknesswriting.com

Ron Kness

Queen Creek, AZ

United States of America

ISBN: 9781653654260

Disclaimer

This publication is for informational purposes only and is not intended as medical advice. Medical advice should always be obtained from a qualified medical professional for any health conditions or symptoms associated with them.

Every possible effort has been made in preparing and researching this material. We make no warranties with respect to the accuracy, applicability of its contents or any omissions.

See your healthcare professional before starting any diet, health or exercise program!

Fitness Game Plan - 2020

Contents

Fitness Game Plan - 2020

Introduction

There is a strange phenomenon that occurs every year just before the New Year. All of a sudden, everyone and their grandmother decides that they're going to get fit and healthy and transform their life.

The fact that they were consuming junk food the entire year and the most exercise they got daily was reaching for the TV remote seems to escape them. These habits that have governed their lives for the most part are given scant regard... because it's a NEW YEAR.

That means it's a new beginning... and a new life awaits them. Right?

Wrong. The road to good health and fitness is littered with the carcasses of those who tried with the best intentions and failed a few weeks into their journey.

Age is just a number

You may have heard the saying, "Age is just a number." Well, in the same vein, 1st January is just a date too. It's no different from August 17 or October 27.

The date you decide to turn your life around has no effect on the chances of you attaining your goals. Step into any gym in January and you'll see it packed to the brim. Step into the same gym in March and it'll be a ghost town.

What happened?

Simple. Reality happened.

You start with a clean slate every day

The truth of the matter is that you are given a clean slate every single day. It doesn't matter whether it's New Year's Day or any other day. What matters is that you make the best of it.

If you've ever made a New Year's resolution to lose weight, and you gave up in February, guess what? All hope is NOT lost.

You can start all over again right now. You have a clean slate every day. Even if you started in August, if you stay on course, you'd lose quite a bit of weight, boost your stamina and increase your strength – if you were on a clean diet and trained daily.

Fitness Game Plan - 2020

You won't need to make a New Year resolution to lose weight again. It's done and dusted. You've achieved your goal.

Focus on increasing the effort, not decreasing the goal

Very often, when people do not attain their goals, they decrease the goals. For example, if they decided to lose 20 pounds and they only managed to lose 3 pounds after one month, they quit and settle for what they got.

You should always focus on increasing the effort. But what if you're giving your best efforts and the results are still abysmal?

The answer is simple, but often overlooked. You just need more time. The more time you give yourself to attain your goal, the cumulative effort expended will be much greater. You did not get overweight and out of shape in a day or two, so why are you fixated on losing weight and getting fit in just a few days?

All things held constant, if you're on track with your diet and training, your efforts multiplied will get you to your goal. Even if you started in March and achieved your goal in September, instead of June like you were hoping for – it doesn't matter. You STILL succeeded.

Give yourself time so that your sweat equity is higher.

Self-discipline is more important than motivation

One reason why most people make resolutions and set goals during New Year's Day is because they feel motivated and inspired. They believe that since it's a new year, they're going to have a new life.

This almost NEVER happens because to get a new life, you'll need to make massive changes to your current mindset and lifestyle. Motivation and inspiration fade very quickly.

Once that happens, you'll need self-discipline to carry you through. You'll find out that there will be days when you just want to quit your diet which is getting on your nerves. There will be days when you want to skip your workouts because they're such an arduous grind.

Fitness Game Plan - 2020

You'll discover that these days often outnumber the days when you feel motivated or inspired to do your best. It's at times like these when you must exercise self-discipline to stay on track to meet your goals.

The term 'self-discipline' almost sounds like a dirty word to those who are used to giving in to their temptations and living life doing whatever they want to do, instead of whatever they need to do.

They fail to realize that no matter how ambitious they feel or how inspired they get on New Year's Day, without self-discipline, they'll be back to square one by February 10th with all their bad habits and actions that lead them nowhere.

You decide when your goal begins and ends

Finally, your goal starts when you decide it starts. You do not need to wait for any day that sounds good. You don't need a New Year's Day or a Monday or a start of a new month, etc.

You can start today, right now… and most winners do. The earlier you start, the faster you'll reach your goal. So why wait?

Your goal ends when it's achieved. If you attain your goal, your journey is over and it's time to make a new goal. Having a deadline is good… but what happens if you reach the deadline and you've still not met your goal?

Will you quit? What if it's December 28th and another New Year is approaching, and you're still stuck with the goal you've not attained yet?

You carry on the struggle till you achieve it. You decide when your goal ends. Not dates, events or other people. Some goals take years to achieve.

Thankfully, health and fitness doesn't require that much time. You can do wonders in 90 days and transform your health completely in 180 days. Even if it takes longer, it's fine.

New Year resolutions are fun… but focus on your daily resolutions. These are the ones that will change your life and take you to heights you never believed you could reach.

Start today; start now. Now that you have made a commitment to get fit in 2020, let's look at some of the things you can do to achieve that goal.

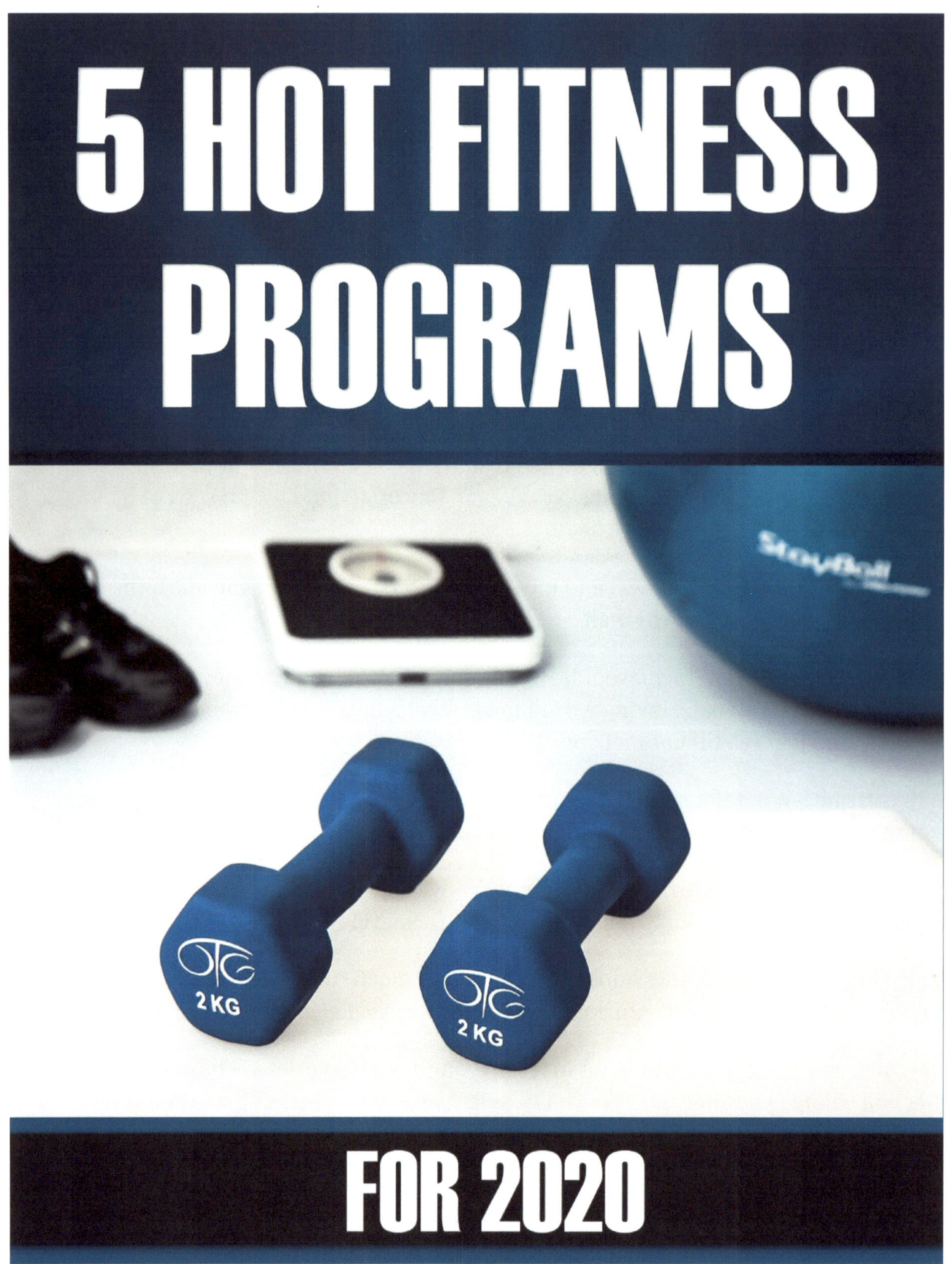
5 HOT FITNESS
PROGRAMS
2 KG
2 KG
FOR 2020

5 Hot Fitness Programs for 2020

If you're trying to figure out which fitness program you should pursue in 2020 to achieve optimal health or another type of fitness goal, you'll be happy to hear there are many options for you to consider.

Five of them are garnering a lot of attention among fitness professionals, their clients and regular gym attendants, making newcomers to the fitness game eager to see what's at the top of their list. You can choose based on your personal preferences and your specific goals.

Bodyweight Exercises for Fitness

Whether you're brand new to fitness or you're a seasoned athlete or fitness buff, bodyweight exercises can be a great way for you to work out if you don't have access to free weights or machines – or, if you don't quite feel ready for them yet.

There are all kinds of bodyweight exercises, ranging from beginner to advanced, and you can really get a full body workout just from doing bodyweight work alone. To start on the easier side, for a good upper body workout you can do pushups.

They're one of the most commonly known bodyweight exercises, but they do work. Depending on how you angle your arms, you can have a more chest intensive workout or a more triceps-intensive one.

You can also adjust your body's angle relative to the floor to make it more or less difficult, depending on what you need. These can be done anywhere, so they make for a perfect upper body exercise using bodyweight.

When it comes to legs, squats are king. Many times, you'll see people doing them with crazy amounts of weight, but bodyweight squats have their purpose, too. By focusing on your form and not the amount of weight you're using, bodyweight squats tend to help you gain the muscle memory you need while also still developing your legs quite a bit.

If you need more difficult variations, you can do things like one-legged squats if you're really strong enough. Pullups are a fantastic exercise for your back, but that doesn't mean they're easy.

Pullups can actually be fairly difficult for some people - especially those who are overweight and not particularly strong. There are all different kinds of grip positions that you can use from things like chin ups to wide grip pull ups, but focus on the standard ones at first before you try to move around too much.

The only downside to pullups is that you do need a stable bar to hold onto that's high up enough for you to pull yourself up with it. For the very advanced fitness enthusiasts, there's a version of the pullup known as a "muscle-up."

Fitness Game Plan - 2020

This involves doing a pull up, getting your whole upper body over the bar, and then pushing yourself up even further by doing a dip. This is a very difficult bodyweight exercise that not a lot of people can do, but if you can, it can do wonders for your strength. No matter what level you're at, bodyweight exercises can always be viable if you adapt them for you.

High Intensity Interval Training for Fitness

High intensity interval training is a fantastic way to both put on muscle and shred down fat. Essentially, you alternate between resting and going as hard as you can for similar amounts of time until you're too tired to do it anymore.

HIIT training, as it's more commonly known, can be done with a variety of exercises, all with different effects and results, so you can experiment a bit to figure out what works best for you.

One of the most common HIIT exercises is sprinting. Many people struggle with running to get in shape, but by doing short bursts of sprinting combined with short periods of rest to catch your breath, you can improve your cardiovascular system, tone your legs, and shed pounds, too.

HIIT allows you to put in a great deal of effort intermittently, instead of putting in a mediocre effort for awhile. This gives you better results with exercises that you might struggle with.

Many people have turned to HIIT in order to get those abs that they've always wanted. By doing extremely intense ab workouts and then resting, you're able to keep going a bit longer than you would with some predetermined sets.

The higher amount of reps means that you're going to see results faster. Much of what makes ab workouts effective for that muscle growth is continuously getting in reps, so with HIIT, you're going to definitely firm up your core.

You can structure your HIIT workouts in different ways. The length of the workout and of each interval can be adjusted to better fit you, though you should be uncomfortable to an extent while doing it.

While some involve exercising and resting, some will have you switch between an easy and a difficult exercise and wait until the end to really rest up. This makes for a very intense workout that's sure to leave you sore the next day.

Not every workout needs to be a HIIT workout. You can do them once a week, once a month, or whatever works for you. Whatever you do, you want to use them to help break up the monotony of standard workouts to confuse your muscles.

Fitness Game Plan - 2020

If you go to the gym and do the same workouts at the same time every week, your muscles will adapt and already be prepared for it, which makes the workout less effective. By throwing HIIT into the mix, your muscles are forced to shake things up.

Crossfit for Fitness

CrossFit has exploded in popularity since the early 2010s. It strays from many of the typical strategies for fitness that you'd typically see in other workout varieties such as bodybuilding or strongman, and even hosts its own competitions to see who's the best at the standard CrossFit exercises.

While it's typically taken in the form of classes at registered CrossFit gyms, you can do a lot of their exercises at any typical gym. The main point of CrossFit is to combine various different kinds of workouts into one routine, while focusing on what's referred to as "functional fitness."

This means that instead of just sticking to weightlifting or running, you do a bit of both and then some more. It's less about seeing how much weight you can lift, and more about building yourself up across the board to be better at handling standard daily things.

Functional fitness means that you're lifting with a purpose. Instead of just trying to look like the strongest person or lift the most on a certain exercise, you're trying to do things that will help you in real life.

You'll be better at moving around, better with balance, and better at using your whole body to do certain things rather than just isolating it to your biceps or legs. For example, if you're lifting a box in real life, you're not just going to use your legs or back or arms.

You're going to use a bit of everything to get the box up easily. CrossFit tends to attract many beginners, because their gyms may be less intimidating than ones that solely focus on lifting weights.

Since it's a class, it's easier for beginners to learn what to do and what not to do. Often, when beginners go to gyms full of people that've been working out for years, they fear that they're going to make a fool out of themselves, and they get inside their own heads for the whole workout.

One of the biggest selling points for CrossFit is that it's just simply more enjoyable. They try to create a fun, engaging environment with a friendly community that allows you to exercise in a way that you'll look forward to. It's less about dragging yourself to the same old gym and waiting for benches to open up and more about seeing what you can manage to do that day in terms of reaching new goals.

Fitness Game Plan - 2020

Yoga and Pilates for Fitness

For many people, when they think of yoga, they think of it as something people do as [meditation](#), a sort of spiritual experience. Others might think of it as just a way to be flexible.

However, once you really get involved with it, you realize just how great it is for your core and for your fitness as a whole. In fact, [yoga](#) is a great way to get in shape while providing you with a variety of other advantages.

The main thing that yoga helps you work out is your core. You might not feel it in some of the beginner positions, but a little later down the line, these exercises can become quite intense.

You'll have to hold a position for minutes at a time that requires a strong core to maintain, almost in the same way that doing planks helps you work out your abs. Naturally, these positions help strengthen your core, but they also help tone it up to make your abs more visible.

It's not just your abs that are benefitting from yoga, though. Given the insane number of poses that you can do in yoga, you'll find that some poses will help your arms, while others will help your legs, and so on.

While yoga isn't the best at building muscle per se, it can help you build strength, and more importantly it can help you tone up your body to reveal the existing muscles that you might have developed outside of yoga.

There are a wide variety of other benefits that you can get from yoga that can help you continue to do other forms of fitness, as well. For example, flexibility is extremely important.

It helps ensure that you're able to do exercises such as squats with proper form, helping reduce injury and increasing the effectiveness of such exercises. Since yoga increases your flexibility, you're able to do weightlifting like this with greater ease.

Another aspect of yoga that helps your fitness is preventing injuries in general. Yoga movements are meant to help your body - specifically your muscles as well as tendons and joints, stay active and prevents them from seizing up.

This helps reduce things like muscle cramps, joint pains, and worse, things like muscle tears or separations. These things can be very painful and are possibly the more dangerous aspects of weightlifting. By doing yoga, you can help prevent these and save yourself the future trouble. However if you do suffer an injury, [learn how](#) to keep training while healing.

Fitness Game Plan - 2020

Strength Training for Fitness

Arguably the most popular form of exercise in fitness is strength training. This involves any and all kinds of weightlifting with the goal of becoming stronger and more muscular. Strength training is a fantastic way to get in shape, and it's the main focus of many people's fitness routines.

For a beginner, it can be a bit intimidating, but you don't need to worry, because it's just as simple as any other form of fitness. The best way to start strength training is to develop a schedule.

Many people do certain body parts on certain days so that they can break it up throughout the week, instead of doing one really long workout that'll tire you out. How you break it up is entirely up to you, but most often you'll see people pairing similar body parts, such as upper body or legs.

One of the most important things to note about strength training is that you should only do the weight that you feel good with. Form is the most important part of weightlifting, so don't try to do some kind of weight that you're not ready for yet.

It's understandable that you might want to make those kinds of advancements sooner rather than later, but take it slow and just trust that you'll get there. Otherwise, you're putting yourself at risk for some pretty serious injuries, or at least some stares from the more experienced members of the gym for doing something silly.

Don't be afraid to ask for help at the gym. So many people tend to get all caught up in their ego that they just try to figure it out for themselves, but sometimes a little bit of help can go a long way.

You're not hiring a personal trainer to walk you through things, unless you want to, but you're just asking for a 30 second piece of advice. It can even help get you somewhat integrated into the gym culture, which might make you feel more comfortable being there.

Be sure to give yourself days to rest between workouts. If you haven't gotten into weightlifting before, you'll soon discover that the day after a good workout you'll be feeling very sore. Don't worry, though.

It's a good sign, meaning that your body's muscles have been worked hard enough that they need to repair. When they do that, they come back larger and stronger, which is what leads to increased strength and increased muscle mass.

Regardless of which fitness program you choose to pursue, including adopting a variety of them, you're bound to see positive results in both a visual and healthy way if you are consistent with it and use proper form.

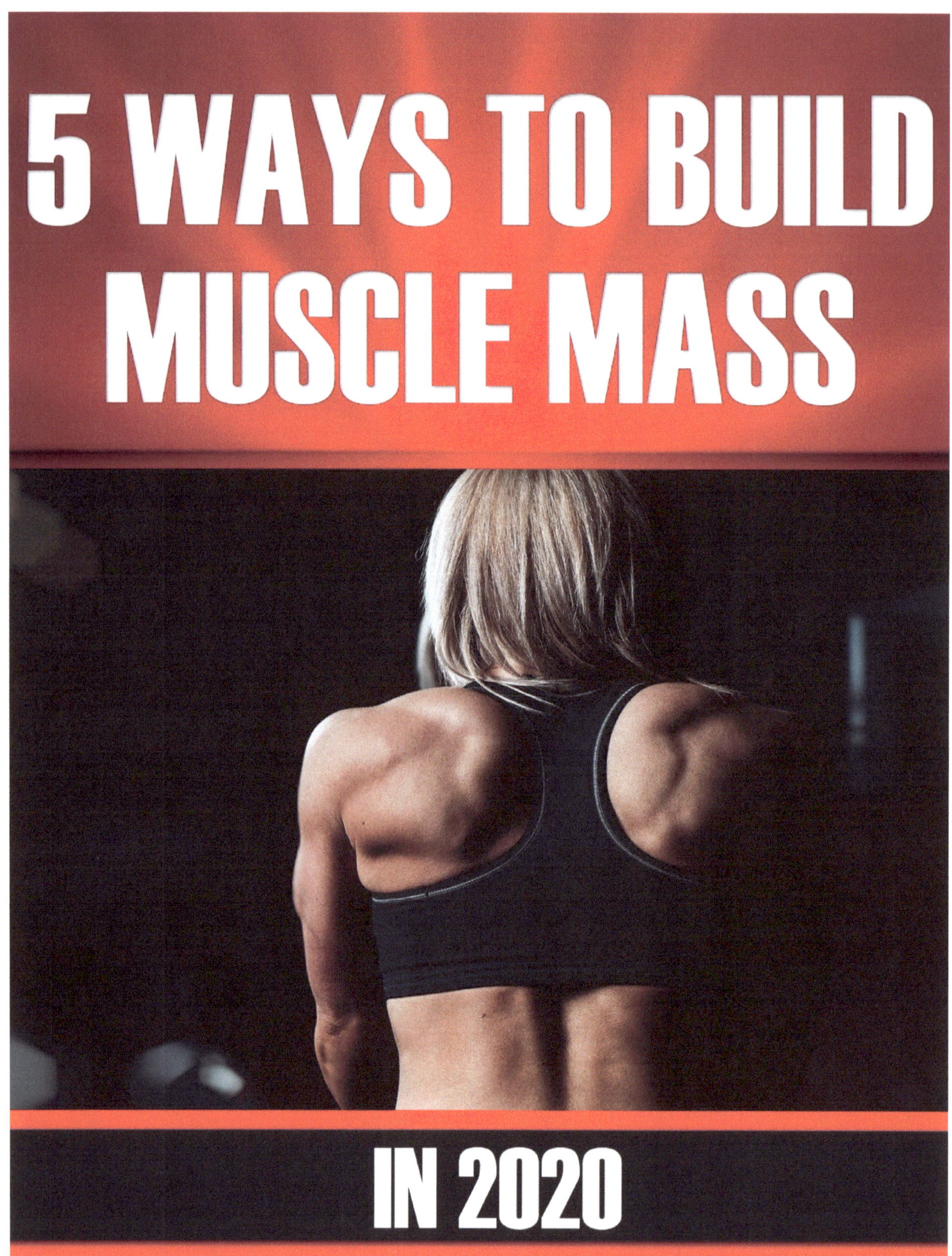
5 WAYS TO BUILD
MUSCLE MASS
IN 2020

5 Ways to Build Muscle Mass in 2020

There's a big difference between toning up and becoming muscular. Building muscle mass takes just as much effort, commitment and patience as losing weight does. Many people think it's only a matter of doing repetitions, but it's more than that.

There are some specific strategies you can incorporate into your fitness routines to help you build muscle mass and bulk up to whatever level you want. It might be just filling your frame out a bit, or really bulking up to a larger-than-life level.

Add Calories You Can Turn into Muscle

Most people's fitness goals are centered around losing weight, because it's very common to have excess fat nowadays. However, there are plenty of people who are actually a bit underweight, and could benefit greatly from putting on some pounds in the form of muscle.

In order to do that effectively, you might have to add some calories to your diet to promote better muscle growth. Just as your body can turn excess calories into fat, you can also turn them into muscle.

When you work out and feel sore afterwards, your body repairs itself using the nutrition from the food you eat in order to create stronger and larger muscles. Having the right nutrition and having enough nutrition is very important for this, because the wrong kinds of calories can leave you without the proper food you need to put on muscles.

Arguably the most important part of your diet for putting on muscles is protein. Proteins are the building blocks of your body, and you need plenty of them for your muscles. Obviously protein can be found in any form of meat, so that's going to be the best initial option for you.

Clean sources of protein like chicken are a staple of many weightlifters' diets, because they provide plenty of protein without things like grease, fat, and extra carbs. If you need a bit of an extra boost, there's always protein shakes.

Protein shakes are a great way to get in a boost of protein after a workout, and they can be made in seconds. Most often you'll see people buy protein powder and mix it into water or milk to make a shake.

Chances are, you're most familiar with whey protein, which specifically helps with muscle growth directly after a workout. This powder comes in all kinds of flavors, so you're sure to find one you like.

There are other supplements that you can take to increase your caloric intake as well. For example, mass gainers are a type of shake similar to protein powder, but with a bunch of other added calories and nutrients to help you put on weight in general.

This can be helpful if you're finding it hard to eat a lot throughout the day, which can be both costly and uncomfortable. By condensing a lot of calories and nutrients into one single shake, your body is more likely to put that mass to use.

Maximize Your Lifts

Many people don't realize that when you go and lift weights, there's a certain strategy to be employed when it comes to how much weight you're doing and how many reps you're doing.

Finding a balance between the two is important, but most people either tend to do high weight with lower reps, or lower weight with high reps. Depending on which one you choose, you can have some drastically different results in terms of how your body looks.

High reps and low weight will get your muscles used to higher amounts of stress and they'll be better adapted for endurance, which is good for things like sports. However, for building muscles, you want to go with higher weight and lower reps.

You might only be able to do five reps with a certain weight but training that way will help you get muscles better than you would with a lower, more comfortable weight. When you lift weights, you're microscopically tearing your muscle fibers.

Not enough to seriously injure you, but this is why you feel sore. When you eat and drink protein, your body repairs those microscopic tears stronger and larger than before to accommodate.

This is how you get stronger and how you build muscles from lifting weights in the first place. By lifting heavier weights, you're putting more direct strain on your muscles rather than testing their endurance, causing more micro-tears, leading to larger muscles.

Lifting heavy is how bodybuilders get into the shape they do, because they solely focus on putting on pure muscle mass while also being sure to shed as much fat as possible, making their muscles pop a bit more.

There's a serious caveat to keep in mind when it comes to heavy lifting: you need to be careful. If you do everything right, you'll put on muscles and keep getting stronger and lifting heavier weight.

However, if you try to lift more weight than you can actually reliably lift, there are going to be some problems. It's not uncommon to see injuries from weightlifting, but most often it comes from people trying to lift as much as humanly possible.

Fitness Game Plan - 2020

You should be aiming for a heavy weight that you can lift for about five reps per set cleanly. If you mess up on your form and have to jerk the weight in a weird way, you can end up causing things like muscles separating from tendons, which can take months, if not years to fully recover.

Stop Getting as Much Cardio

Those who aren't very familiar with fitness will sometimes lump a bunch of exercises with very different purposes together and just call it "working out." This is commonly seen with cardio being lumped together with weightlifting.

If you want to put on muscle mass and gain weight, then you really don't need to be doing much cardio, because it could actually be doing you more harm than good in terms of your goals.

When you do cardio, your body uses up its energy pretty quickly before going to reserves. It'll use fat, which is why it's good for people who want to lose weight. However, those are people with excess fat.

If you're underweight and don't have much fat on you, it'll actually start using up bits of muscle mass, because that provides energy for your body just the same. Instead, you need to focus more of your time on weightlifting, which will increase your muscle mass rather than reduce it.

You might've noticed that in things like sports, there are a lot of different body types depending on the athletes. Runners are almost always skinny and barely have any muscle mass on them, with the exception of definition in their legs.

Someone like a wrestler, on the other hand, will have a lot more fat, but also a lot more muscle. For most people, the ideal body is muscular, but not to the point where you look unnatural, and cut down enough so that your muscles are visible and you don't have excess flab.

If you're starting from a point of already being underweight, you probably don't need many adjustments in terms of body fat percentage - you just need to put on more muscle.

It almost seems counterintuitive that not working out in one way can help you get a better physique, but it's true. Focusing on weightlifting alone also makes things less complicated for your schedule, so you don't have to figure out a cardio day and a weightlifting day - just know when you're going to go lift.

If you still want to keep your cardio in good shape, it's recommended that you do high intensity, fast burst of cardio like sprints and circuits rather than doing something like long steady runs. This helps reduce the amount of energy that your body takes away, and can also help you develop some good leg muscles while keeping your heart healthy.

Take Supplements to Help Build Mass

Getting enough food to sustain mass growth just isn't feasible in some cases. You need a lot of calories to gain weight - especially with a high metabolism, so you'd have to be practically force feeding yourself in order to put on weight effectively.

Not to mention, it also costs more and takes more time to keep eating throughout the day. In order to save time and money, you should incorporate supplements into your daily routine.

It's much easier to fit calories in as fluids, since they don't crowd your stomach quite as much as solid food would. For this reason, many have turned towards meal supplement shakes as a way to put on weight.

You can combine a ton of different foods into some basic shakes and get a great calorie dense meal without breaking the bank or wasting time cooking. Along with supplements, you'll be set to go.

The most common supplement is mass gainer. It comes as a simple powder, usually with some kind of sweet flavor, and it is loaded with nutrients. A single scoop of the stuff can contain as many calories as a typical meal, loaded up with all kinds of carbs, fats, and proteins that you need in order to gain weight.

In one shake, you could have two meals worth of calories without the cost or stomach pains of eating two meals. People often don't just drink their shakes with mass gainer alone.

You can combine it with something like protein powder, which has fewer calories, but bumps up your protein intake a bunch. This kind of shake would be perfect right after a workout to help you recover efficiently and retain all that progress you made at the gym.

You can also mix in foods to your shake if you use a blender, which is highly recommended. People have mixed in fruits, peanut butter, yogurt, and more to give themselves a better tasting shake with more nutrients, so you can really make just about whatever you'd like.

For example, you could take chocolate flavored mass gainer and blend it with milk and some strawberries, giving you a chocolate-covered strawberry shake. Before a workout, if you're more advanced, you might consider supplements such as creatine or pre-workouts in order to help further the growth of muscle building. These products can have health hazards in some people, so be sure to carefully read the packaging to make sure it's safe for you to take it.

Fitness Game Plan - 2020

Let Sleep Help You Build More Muscle

Gaining muscle isn't all about working out. You can lift every single hour of every single day and you will gain muscle, just not as much as you could be. In order for you to gain muscle, you need to tear your muscles microscopically first.

This is what you're doing when you're lifting heavy weights. However, those tears get repaired by your body using protein and a variety of other molecules, leading to muscle mass increasing, along with strength.

So, while you might get those microscopic tears in the first place, if you're not recovering properly, you won't see the full benefits of the growth. Recovery is so important for building muscle, which is why many people have rest days in between workouts.

However, one of the most important stages of recovery is proper sleep. When you're asleep, your body is doing quite a bit of work. Specifically, your muscles are keeping themselves busy by repairing whatever damage you might've done to them throughout the day or during a workout.

Your blood flow to your muscles goes up quite a lot while you're sleeping, and during that time the blood is carrying along key nutrients that your muscles will use to grow and recover.

This is the point in time where that protein you drink and that food you eat is going to get put to use. Your body even naturally produces some HGH, or human growth hormone, which some people take excessively and artificially like steroids.

These hormones are crucial to helping your muscles build up, so proper amounts of sleep are very important to making sure you're healing up properly. You should be getting around eight hours of sleep per night.

This gives your body enough time to go through all of the necessary stages of sleep, including the stage that involves muscle recovery and growth. If you cut off your sleep early, you might not reach that stage, leaving you still feeling sore the next morning.

Find a way to fit proper amounts of sleep in your schedule, no matter what. If you don't sleep enough, not only will you not see an increase in muscle mass, but you'll also have weaker lifts.

If you're not well rested when you go to work out, your body isn't going to have prepared itself enough to reliably get working. If you want to see yourself lift heavier weight and put on more muscle, get to bed earlier and wake up on time.

As you embark on your mission to gain muscle mass, keep track of what works and expand on that rather than completely switching gears or giving up. You might see some gains with increased calories, for example, so if you want to gain more, you may have to eat even more.

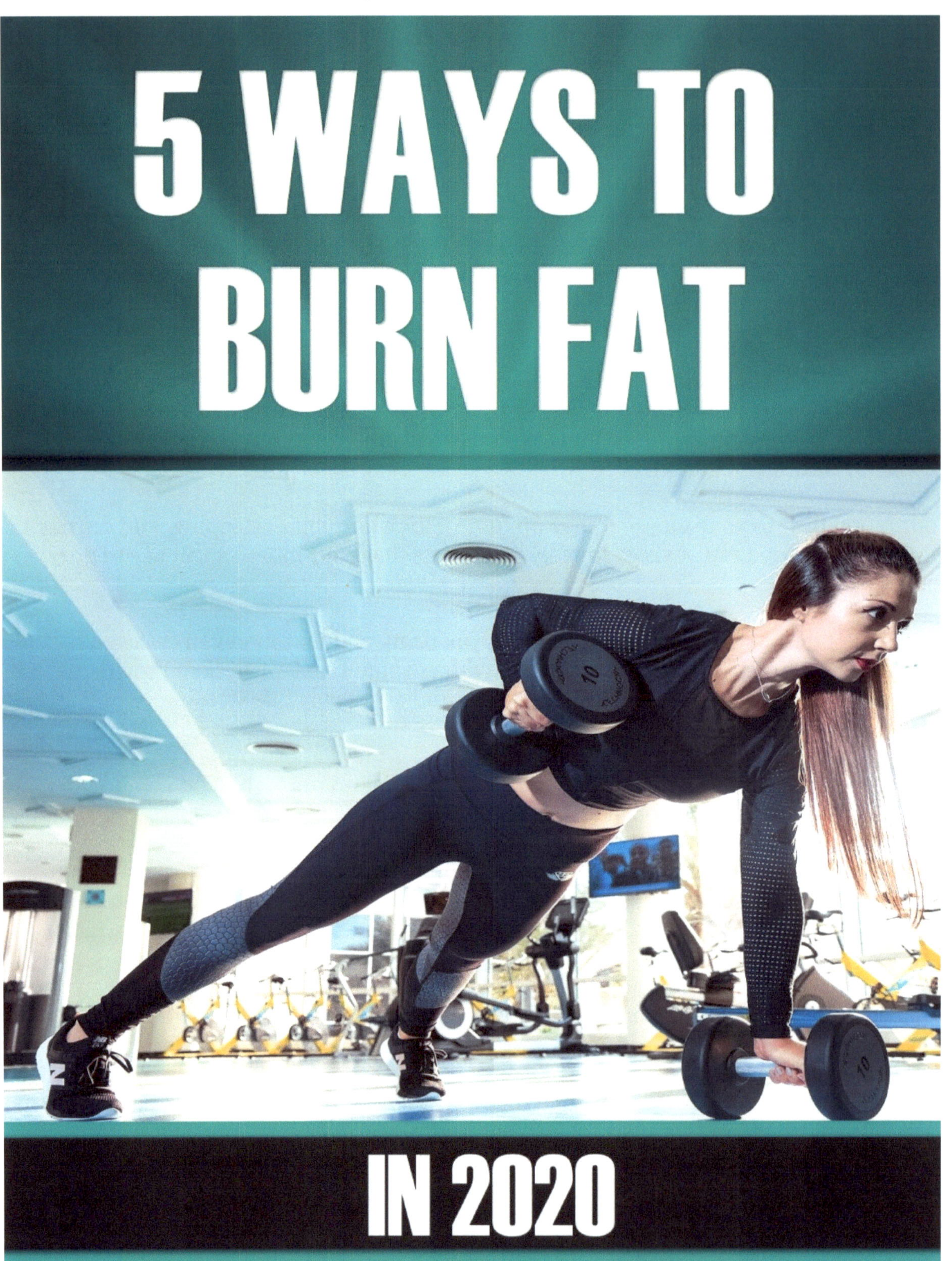

5 WAYS TO
BURN FAT
IN 2020

5 Ways to Burn Fat in 2020

When it comes to looking good and feeling great, fat is the ball and chain that can derail those efforts. You can work out and tone the muscles in your stomach, for example, but unless you burn the fat on top of it, no one will see those six pack abs.

There are many ways to burn fat, but you need to find something that works well for you – something that's easy for you and that you enjoy so you can have some consistency with it.

Use Cardio to Fight Fat Quickly

The main goal of most people's fitness is to simply lose weight. Many people today are overweight, and it's almost always due to the amount of fat they keep on them. There are plenty of options out there that you can use in order to fight fat and get yourself back to looking thin, but the most common one is certainly cardio.

In just about any gym you go into, you'll find that they have rows and rows of cardio equipment. Whether it be treadmills, ellipticals, stair climbers, or anything else, they'll have cardio machines there because they're in high demand.

Running and other forms of cardio are fantastic both for burning off fat and making your heart healthier and more efficient. The reason it's called cardio is that it's a shortened version of the term "cardiovascular," meaning something related to the heart.

Your cardiovascular health is your heart health, for example. When you run and do cardio, your heart rate goes up, and practicing that with consistency over a period of time means that your heart will continue to get stronger and stronger, with increased blood flow and an overall healthier body.

Cardio helps you fight fat by using up stored sources of energy to keep you going as you get tired. Your body uses two different things for energy. First, it uses carbohydrates, or carbs for short.

This is the most baseline energy source for your body because it's the most efficient. However, your body will also use fat, because fat is there to act as storage for energy in the event that it's needed later down the line.

In order to get the best results out of using cardio for fat burn, you should combine it with a lower-carb diet. This means that your body will have to go through less carbs and will start using fat as fuel sooner, making the time between starting cardio and fat burn shorter than it would be on a normal diet.

There are tons of ways to get cardio in, whether it be in a very formal fashion or one that's more enjoyable. Many people stick with treadmills or exercise bikes, but there are so many other good options.

You can go hiking, go on long walks if the weather is nice, swim at an indoor pool, and so much more. No matter what you like to do, there's going to be a form of cardio out there for you.

Let Strength Training Help You Burn Fat Faster

Burning fat isn't solely based on cardio. While many people think of weightlifting and strength training as just a way to build muscle, it's actually a good way to burn off fat as well if you do it right.

There are tons of benefits with strength training that will help you burn fat, build muscle, and look more toned very quickly. There's a big difference in strength training between high reps and low reps.

This is basically referring to the amount of repetitions you do in each set of your workout. For example, if someone was doing 3 sets of bench press, there's a big difference in doing 3 sets of 15 reps and 3 sets of 5 reps.

Naturally you'd change the weight you're using to do more or less reps, but it does different things for your body. When you do heavy weights and low reps, you're making your body stronger.

Your body becomes more used to the high amount of pressure and the work it takes to move that weight, but it doesn't help you much in the weight loss department. Doing low weight and high reps doesn't make you as strong, but it's much better at helping you put on muscle mass and burning fat.

When you're doing high reps, you'll probably be a bit sweaty and out of breath after the last few reps. This is a great sign. If you're sweating, you're burning calories. It takes a lot of energy out of your body to continuously move weight like that, so in a very similar vein to cardio, your body has to use fat as a source of such energy.

One major benefit of strength training is that, unlike cardio, it's purely taking away fat as a source of energy. If you do nothing but cardio, you'll get thin, but you won't have much muscle on you, as cardio can burn muscle a bit on its own.

By doing strength training, you'll still lose the fat, but you won't have to sacrifice any muscle. In fact, you'll be building up muscle, giving you the strong, toned look that you want much faster.

Fitness Game Plan - 2020

Strength training can help you focus on areas that are problem spots for you. In cardio, you're losing weight equally across your whole body. With strength training, you can pick exercises that only target certain areas. For example, with stomach fat, you can focus on core workouts, or tricep workouts for things like excessive fat on underarms.

Use Protein to Reduce Fat in Your Body

Many people's weight problems today stem from their diets. The average diet is predominately carbs, followed by fats, and then in last, protein. This would be normal for someone who's working out constantly like an Olympic athlete, but for the average person, this diet leads to a lot of issues - the main one being weight gain.

What a lot of people don't understand about nutrition is that carbs are our fuel source, but they have to be used when you eat them. The worst thing that you can do is eat a lot of carbs and then sit around doing nothing, because you'll have all that fuel go to waste.

What your body then does is create fat deposits to store that energy in case you need it later, leaving you with excess fat and more weight. Carbs come in plenty of forms, from sweets to sodas to bread.

Some are better than others, but none of them are great if you're not using them enough. Instead, you'll want to replace some of your carbs with proteins. Protein is what your body uses predominantly to build itself up, specifically in terms of muscle.

While this doesn't mean that you'll magically gain muscle from eating protein, your muscles will be less prone to injury and will not get as sore as they would on a low-protein diet.

You want to make sure you don't lose all your carbs, because just by existing your body needs some fuel to keep going. However, just substitute out the unnecessary amounts with protein to get a more balanced diet.

There are plenty of great sources of protein out there for anyone to enjoy. The most common one for a lot of people is meat. This means things like beef and pork, but more importantly things like chicken or turkey.

While red meat does provide a good amount of protein, it's often accompanied by fats and other macros, or it's paired with carbs. Take, for example, a burger, which does have red meat, but is also filled with things like bread and cheese and condiments that make it less healthy.

For a healthy meat-based source of protein, you want to look towards poultry and fish. Chicken and turkey provide sources of lean meat, meaning that they're low in fat but high in protein. These can be paired with things like salads to make for a great, healthy lunch that will improve your protein intake.

Fitness Game Plan - 2020

Increase Your Fiber Intake to Shed Fat Swiftly

Fiber is an often overlooked nutrient that you need from your food. People tend to get so caught up in the calories and the macros of their diets that they forget about all the other things that go into getting a healthy meal.

Fiber helps your body in many ways, but one of the most beneficial is in terms of weight loss. Specifically, fiber has been shown to help people lose and keep off belly fat, which is one of the worst kinds of fat health-wise.

One way that fiber helps you burn fat is by bettering your gut health. Inside your digestive system, you have an expansive network of bacteria that is extremely important for you to survive.

These bacteria help you break food down and digest it properly, so it's important to have the right array of them there. For some people, their gut bacteria may be low or all very similar, meaning that they can have problems fully digesting their foods.

Fiber has been shown to help diversify your digestive bacteria, which can help quite a bit with weight loss. One of the best ways that fiber helps you lose fat is simply by making you less hungry.

Some people eat whether they're hungry or not, but a lot of people also just have a big appetite. By naturally suppressing your hunger, fiber helps you eat less, meaning that you'll have a better calorie deficit, leading to fantastic weight loss.

There are plenty of great sources of fiber out there. In most stores, you can simply find fiber pills, which can give you most of your daily dose of fiber. This is for those that can't really adapt to a new diet, but still want to experience some of the benefits of more fiber.

These pills are fairly inexpensive, and you can get plenty of fiber easily. However, the healthier way of increasing your fiber intake would be to slowly up the amount you're getting over time, so that your body can adjust as needed.

This would be from making little changes in your diet here and there by adding in things like oatmeal or certain vegetables. If you're not used to fiber, a sudden influx of it can lead to a few minor digestive problems. Nothing dangerous, but nonetheless uncomfortable. If done right, though, fiber can be a great contributing factor to your weight loss.

Cut Carbs to Shape Up and Say Goodbye to Fat

Carbs are one of the largest contributors to weight and fat gain for most people today. So many foods are absolutely loaded with unhealthy carbs that cause your weight to skyrocket, and it ends up being very detrimental to your health for a number of reasons.

Fitness Game Plan - 2020

In order to effectively get rid of fat, you need to adjust your carb intake quite a bit. The reason carbs cause you to gain weight is that, when going unused, your body creates fat deposits and stores them there for another time.

They also tend to be accompanied by high amounts of calories, which, if you're not burning them off, will naturally cause weight gain by giving you a greater amount of calories in than out.

One common misconception is that since carbs cause weight gain, you should cut them out altogether. In reality, that can lead to a few complications and is not advisable. Carbs are a very important part of your body's natural cycle to produce energy.

Carbohydrates, such as sugar, have glucose which your body uses to create ATP, the molecule responsible for just about everything you do. It allows your muscles to move, your mind to think, and so on.

However, your body doesn't need a ton of it to keep you going throughout the day. Instead of cutting out carbs altogether, you just need to cut back on the amount you're consuming.

There's plenty of foods that you might be eating that contain an insane amount of unnecessary carbs. One of the greatest offenders in modern society is soda. An average single can of soda contains upwards of 40 grams of sugar, a very common carb.

This amount is about twice what you would need to simply sustain yourself throughout the day. With people drinking multiple cans or even glasses of this drink per day, it's no wonder weight gain is so common.

Cut out any and all sweet and sugary drinks in order to make some serious progress towards weight loss. Other common suspects include fast food, which is cooked in very high carb breading and oils, as well as sweets.

These are foods that people typically think of when dieting, but there are lesser known high carb foods out there as well. Foods like potatoes, bread, and pasta are high carb and typically not considered to be unhealthy, but they can certainly lead to fat gain just as any other high carb food can.

Keep in mind that if you ever get to a point where the fat isn't burning as fast as you'd like it to, you can swap things up and implement a new strategy to kickstart the fat burning process after a plateau.

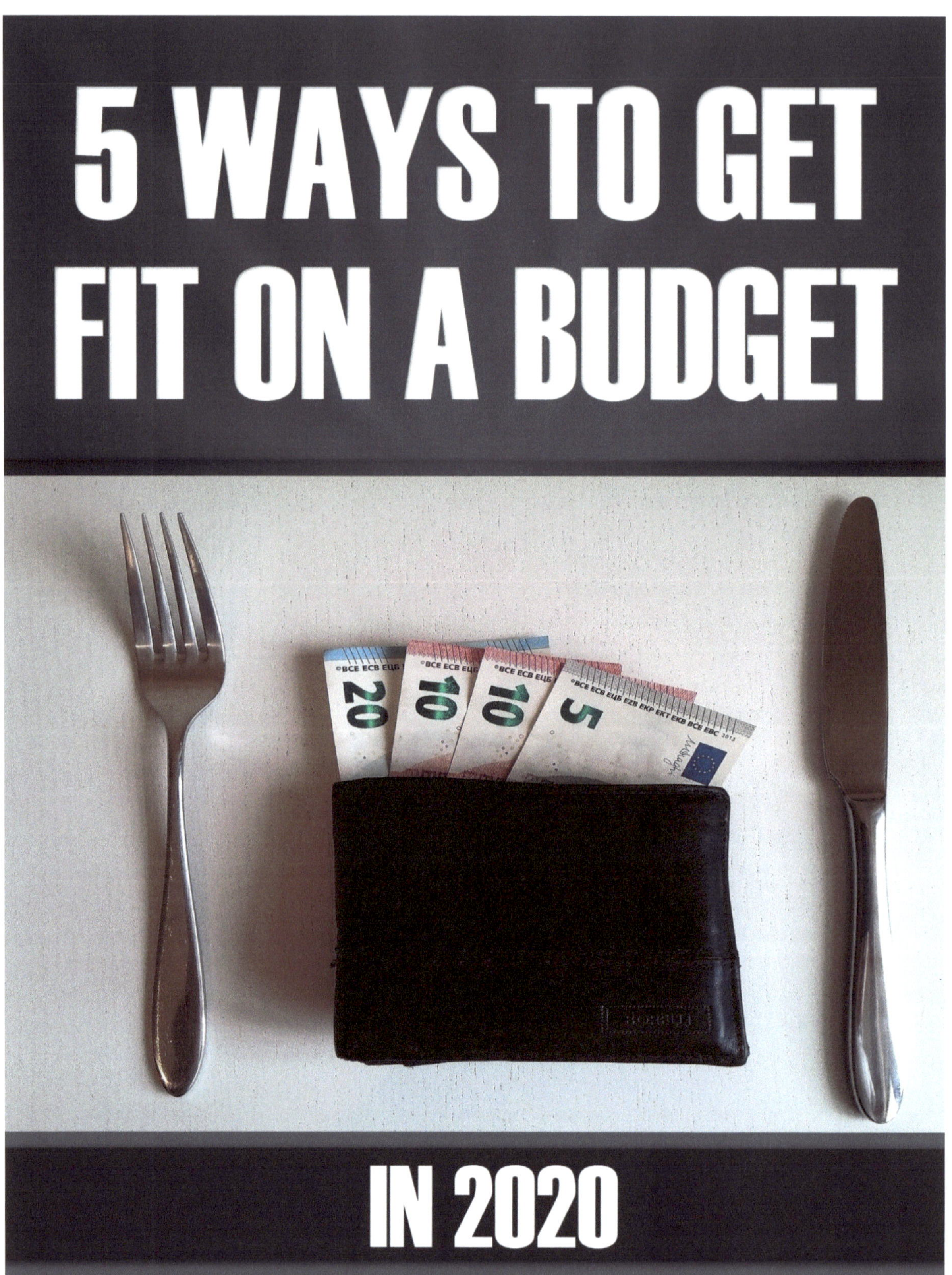
5 WAYS TO GET
FIT ON A BUDGET
IN 2020

5 Ways to Get Fit on a Budget In 2020

Getting fit can sometimes be a financial burden to many people – or at least, that's what they think. We often hear how good, clean foods are most expensive and we know a gym membership, personal training and equipment is sometimes out of our price range.

At times, price is used as an excuse, but if you're serious about achieving your fitness goals, then you won't allow anything to stand in your way. You can achieve any fitness goal you set for yourself on any type of budget – big or small.

Build a Home Gym on the Cheap

Getting a gym membership can be costly. If there's not a cheap gym near you, you can be paying quite a bit of money per month to have access to the gym. Even then, it may not be a 24-hour gym, so you have to work with their hours to get your workout in on time.

Building a home gym saves you a lot of money in the long run, but it doesn't have to be expensive at the start anyway. People are sometimes put off by home gyms because the equipment can get expensive if you buy it new.

Things like treadmills can cost hundreds of dollars, and weightlifting machines can cost even more. Gyms can afford them because they have hundreds of people paying for memberships, but you're just one person.

Instead of buying all of your equipment new, look towards the secondhand market. It's not uncommon for people to sell exercise equipment or even give it away because they'll try to build up a home gym and then give up on it, leaving them with these items that are taking up space.

You can find all kinds of essentials using websites like eBay or Craigslist, and usually for a much better price than you'd find brand new. It's also important that you don't buy equipment that you don't need.

Certain things like machines that drive up the cost of a home gym aren't really necessary if you can learn how to do those exercises with free weights - meaning things like dumbbells and barbells.

They almost always have a free weight counterpart, so you only need to buy those. A good set of dumbbells can be acquired for just around $250 or less, and those can be used for just about any kind of workout and will get you in shape.

That's if you decide to get a set with different kinds of dumbbells going up to around 50 pounds. If you want an even cheaper option, you can get an adjustable dumbbell, which allows you to use one pair of them and change the weight through a wide range.

Fitness Game Plan - 2020

This helps save space and money. Another good essential to get is a bench and barbell. Naturally, this allows you to do bench press, which is a common exercise, but it also enables you to do things like overhead press and squats, all for next to nothing. A bench is almost always less than $50, and a barbell can be picked up for around $20.

Use Natural Fitness Regimens

Not every exercise requires the use of a gym or gym equipment. There are many fitness regimens that can be done with nothing but your body, and it's often more enjoyable that way.

Exercising naturally can get you in shape without you having to spend a dime on things like gym memberships or at-home equipment. The first thing that you don't need any kind of membership for is running.

People tend to like using treadmills, but going outside and running is just as viable. Hopefully, you live in an area with fairly nice weather, where it's not too hot, too cold, or too rainy to get out and run.

If so, pick up some running shoes, some earbuds, and go on a run around your city or neighborhood. Running outdoors is much more enjoyable than staring at the wall with a treadmill.

Next, there are plenty of exercises that don't require you to use weights. For example, squats are often seen being done with a barbell and plates loaded up on it, but that's not necessary for a beginner.

Bodyweight squats are going to help you work out your legs just as well as anything else - you just need to increase the amount of reps you're doing. Similarly, you can work out your chest and triceps by doing pushups with proper form.

This removes the need to go out and get something like a bench for bench press. By changing the angle of your elbows and the elevation of your body, you can make pushups easier or harder to account for your skill level.

There are also tons of things that you can do throughout your day-to-day life in order to be a bit more active. They may seem small, but they add up over time. For example, when you go to a store or to work, you probably try to pick the closest parking spot that you can.

Try parking further back - it'll make your walk longer, but that's helping you get in more steps. Similarly, whenever you have to go to a second or third floor in a building, take the stairs instead of an elevator or escalator. This can help get you a bit of a leg workout and it also helps get you some cardio. This alone isn't going to get you in shape, but it helps you more than you might think.

Fitness Game Plan - 2020

Shop in Grocery Stores - Not for Fad Diet Foods

Something that helps a lot both for your budget and for your health is buying food from the grocery store and cooking for yourself. It's such a simple change, but many people don't do it.

It can save you hundreds per month and, if you do it right, you'll be losing weight in no time thanks to the healthier options provided there. Fast food is just horrible for you. It's always going to be loaded with grease, salt, fat, and excess carbs, which are all bad news if you're trying to lose weight.

It can also be costly, being around $7 for a meal. In comparison, meals made at home typically cost you about $1-2. Over time, this adds up quite a lot of savings. Before heading to the store, make sure you have recipes with ingredient lists so that you know exactly what you need to get and how much of it you need to get.

This helps you avoid walking around lost, grabbing random things and trying to make a healthy meal out of it. Once you have all the ingredients you need, you're good to go. One of the things that you might have tried before while shopping is buying some fad dieting products.

Things that claim to help you lose weight fast in the form of diet pills, frozen diet meals, brand diet plans or meal replacement shakes. Sometimes it'll be a particular food that people are claiming to have "magical weight loss effects."

Don't buy into these, because they're really not as trustworthy as they might seem. When it comes to diet and weight loss, if it seems too good to be true, it probably is. Chances are slim that there's really a product that's going to help you drop 30 pounds in 2 weeks.

While we don't like accepting this fact, it's true - weight loss takes time, effort, and commitment. Instead of wasting your money gambling on some weight loss scam product, go with tried and true methods.

Eating smaller, healthier meals will cause you to lose weight, and that's been proven time after time. Just because one person claims to have dropped a ton of weight after taking some pill doesn't mean it's going to be true – or long lasting.

Buying groceries and cooking at home is not only a more affordable option, but it's also one that will help you get in shape and will give you some more variety in your meals, leading to an overall happier life.

Use Digital Media to Guide Your Workout

People are often hesitant to get in shape because they're unsure of what to do and believe that they need to hire a personal trainer and other similar professionals in order to have a successful attempt at fitness.

Fitness Game Plan - 2020

In this day and age with the internet, that's simply not true. You can find everything you need and more using digital media - you just need to know where to look. The first problem people tend to run into is not having a workout plan.

You might have stepped into a gym before and felt totally lost. You don't know what machines to use, how to use them, and haven't even considered touching the free weight area.

All you really know are dumbbell curls and maybe a few things for your legs. At this point, some people think of hiring a personal trainer to tell them what to do, but that can be out of some people's price range.

Instead, look online at workout forums. Most of them have beginner guides with detailed information about what to do in order, how much of it you should do, what to look for, and so on.

You can save it on your phone or jot it down and head to the gym with a perfect guide, saving you from the embarrassment of just meandering around the gym. Another great resource for workout tips is YouTube.

Through YouTube, you can find quick and easy visual guides on workouts that you don't quite know how to do. A lot of the terminology can get confusing, and trying to describe some workouts in words can be difficult.

If you don't have a friend or a personal trainer to show you what to do, people on YouTube can tell you in just around a minute, and they'll give you some useful tips as well.

You should also look to digital media for diet planning. You don't need to go and pay for sessions with a nutritionist to tell you what you should be eating. There are so many people that catalogue their full meals online with recipes all the time.

Following other people's meal plans can get you the same results that they're seeing, and you don't have to spend a dime for someone to tell you what to eat. Finally, you can download apps on your smart phone to help you tracks your workout progress. There are apps that help you with everything from workout routines to diet tracking, and you should use them to help your fitness progress.

Join a Local Adult Sports Team

Sometimes, the best way to get in shape isn't to join an expensive gym or buy a bunch of equipment, but rather to just spend some good time playing sports. Chances are, you have an adult sports team in your area that you could have a good time with.

These teams are a great way to get in shape at a low cost. First, they provide you with a way to get in your cardio. For most people, this is what they're missing for their fitness.

Fitness Game Plan - 2020

Whether you're playing soccer, baseball, basketball, skating, or anything else, you're probably going to be spending a lot of time running or at least doing some kind of intensive cardio.

This is much different from cardio at the gym, though. At the gym, you'd run on a treadmill or an elliptical. This is a pretty boring movement that you repeat ad nauseam until you feel like you've done enough.

If you're lucky, they might have TVs that you can watch, but if not, you're just staring at the wall or at the rest of the gym. In sports, on the other hand, you're doing varied movements that help keep your body more limber and dynamic, and you're not as likely to get bored.

Instead of just using your legs and walking, you might be using your arms, ducking down, moving side to side, and so on. This makes the workout much more interesting, and time flies fast so it doesn't feel like you've been walking forever.

Another thing joining a team like this does for you is hold you accountable. If you don't really feel like going to the gym, and you don't have a gym partner or anything like that, you're just not going to go.

However, if a team is counting on you to be there, you're going to be much more likely to show up whether you feel like it or not, because you're being held accountable. It's really nice to be able to spend time with new people and do something that you enjoy.

Gyms can get stagnant and boring after some time. It's much more enjoyable to do something that varies and changes and helps you grow as a person. Combined with the fact that team dues are cheaper than a gym membership, it's a really great alternative to working out - especially if you're on a budget.

Remember, you can always find a way to achieve fitness goals – whether it's weight loss, building muscle mass, improving mobility or range of motion, or more. It doesn't matter how much or how little you have to spend on this pursuit.

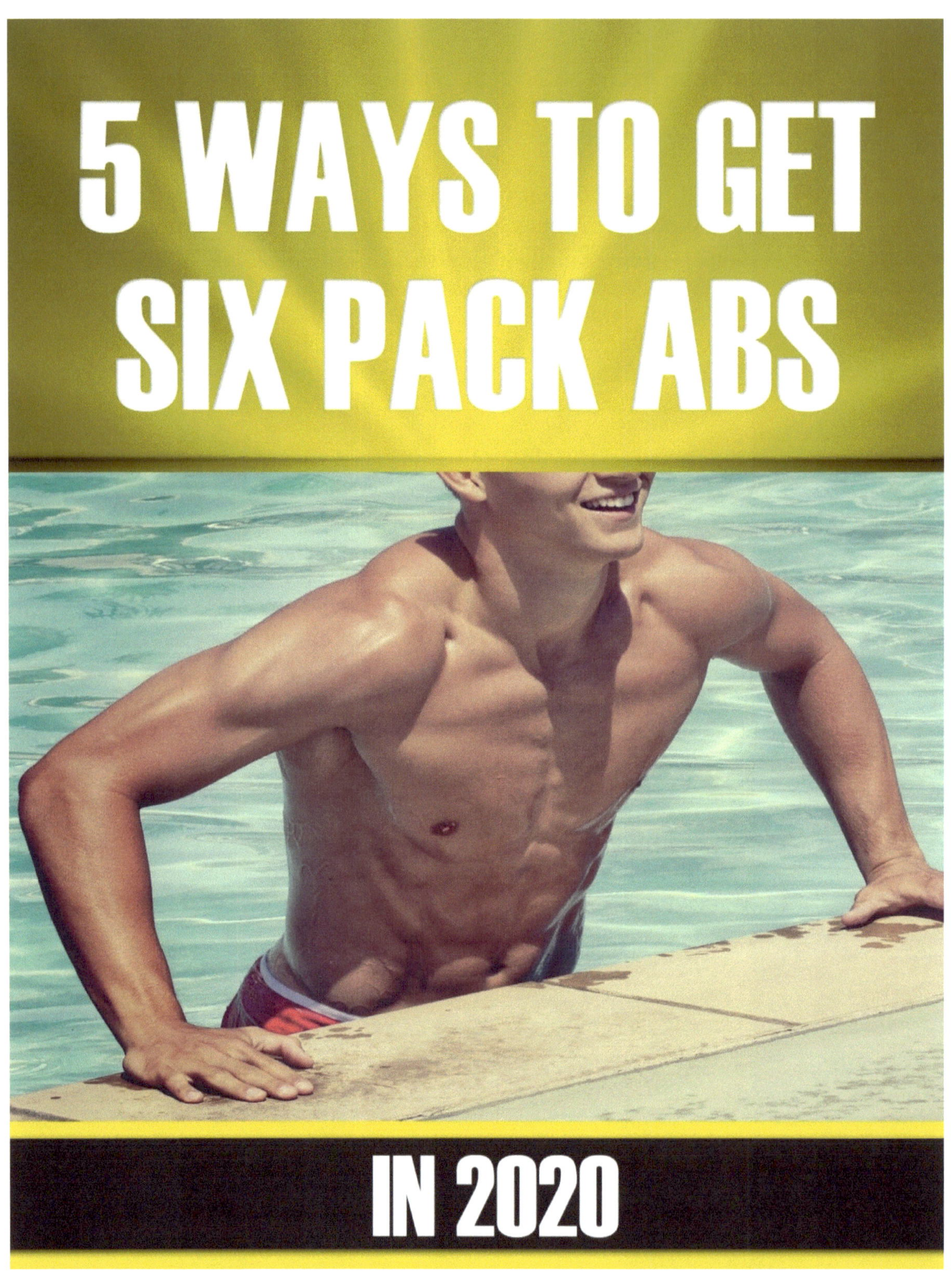

5 WAYS TO GET
SIX PACK ABS
IN 2020

5 Ways to Get Six Pack Abs in 2020

One of the ultimate ways to showcase your fitness is by showing off your six-pack abs. It's become a common badge of honor among fitness enthusiasts to be able to prove that they have them.

There are many things you can do to shed fat and reveal the toned and carved ab muscles you want everyone to see – or just for your own personal satisfaction! Sometimes it has nothing to do with showcasing anything, and everything to do with simply feeling strong and healthy.

Increase Cardio to Tone Your Tummy

When people think about what they'd look like being in shape, one of the most commonly sought after features is having six pack abs. Everyone wants abs because it's seen as a pinnacle in fitness, meaning that not only do you have a flat stomach, but you've also toned and worked it out to where the abs can shine through.

There are a lot of steps to get to that point, one of which is using cardio to tone up your midsection. For many people, their lack of abs is from a combination of excess fat hiding them as well very little (if any) definition from a lack of exercise.

This is why cardio is a great starting point to work towards them. Cardio helps you burn fat, but it also engages your core along with your legs, helping you develop muscles there so that you can see your abs a bit faster to begin with.

There are some forms of cardio that just happen to work better than others for this purpose. For example, rowing machines and jumping rope force you to engage your abs more, making them more defined.

Things like swimming are mostly for burning belly fat. It's not a really massive difference, so as long as you're doing a form of cardio you enjoy, that's what matters. As far as scheduling goes, you should be doing cardio around 3 times a week.

Whether you combine it with your weightlifting days or keep them separate is up to you, though many people prefer to keep them separate so they're not too tired to do either the weightlifting or the cardio.

At that rate, you'll be in a pretty good spot to start developing some abs. It's also helpful to mix up the cardio you're doing not only so that you don't get bored, but also to hit slightly different parts of the body.

Not every form of cardio attacks belly fat in the exact same way, so by mixing things up, you're more likely to see results instead of letting things get stagnant. Do a different form of cardio each time you go throughout the week or alternate each week if you like settling in a bit longer.

If there's one thing to remember, though, it's that no matter how much cardio you do, diet is still going to be important. Your intense cardio session can be undone in a single meal, so plan your diet carefully if you really want those abs.

Engage in Specific Ab Building Exercises

One of the most important parts of having a six pack is actually building your abs up. They don't usually just appear when you've lost enough weight - they're muscles just like any other and they need to be exercised.

By doing core workouts, you'll be able to see your abs faster and you'll give yourself a few other benefits along the way. Ab workouts tend to be fairly straightforward. The most common one that people tend to recognize from gym class is the sit-up.

Sit-ups are decent ab exercises, but they don't give you quite the same benefits that you might get doing some other, more effective ones. You need someone or something to keep your feet down if you can't do that naturally, and sometimes they're a bit too easy.

Instead, one of your main ab exercises should be crunches. Crunches are similar to sit-ups, but a bit more comfortable in some ways, and you see just as good of results, if not better.

Instead of balancing on your tailbone and pulling up your whole upper body, you lay flat and bring up your body just a bit while also pulling in your legs. This helps work out your abs, but it's a lot better for your back than sit-ups are.

While many people often don't like doing them, planks are a fantastic ab exercise. If you haven't done them before, they're actually quite simple. You get into an almost push-up like form, but instead of having your hands down, you lay your elbows and forearms flat in front of you.

Keeping your back straight and your knees off the ground, you just hold that position for around a minute. This puts a ton of stress on your core and will definitely get you the results you want.

Some of the more fun types of ab workouts are those that involve medicine balls. Medicine balls are those weighted balls you find in the gym that are rubbery and dense. They usually weigh between 2 and 10 pounds, and are typically basketball sized or smaller.

Fitness Game Plan - 2020

With these, you can do tons of ab workouts that are a bit more enjoyable since you're at least doing something. One great one, if your gym allows it and has space for it, is combining crunches with medicine ball tosses.

Basically, you do crunches with your feet up against the wall, and when you come up, you toss the medicine ball and have it bounce off back into your hands and repeat. This helps break up the monotony of just a standard crunch workout.

Alter Your Diet to Shed Fat That's Hiding Your Abs

The most important part of getting abs to begin with is the diet. You can work out your abs every day and not see them unless you get rid of the belly fat that's covering them up.

Belly fat is a common, yet dangerous kind of fat, being linked to heart disease among other things. It hides your abs in such a way that people only really see a gut or a bit of flab there, even if you have abs underneath.

In order to show off your abs, you need to adjust your diet in such a way that you'll lose that belly fat. Now everyone's diet is certainly different, but there are fairly common things that you can try that will likely help you reduce the amount of belly fat you have so that you can better see your abs.

First, cutting sugary, liquid calories is a must. This mostly includes sodas. Sodas are one of the least healthy things you can consume and will cause rapid gain of belly fat. They're absolutely full of empty calories and contain an insane amount of carbs, and that's in one can alone.

Often times, people will get a large cup full of it, which is easily a meal's worth of carbs and calories all by itself. Next, you should obviously avoid unnecessary sweets. It's tempting to want to eat dessert, but if you can find a healthier option like fruits or low calories sweets, go for those.

Desserts are often chock full of sugar, meaning they're going to go straight to your belly as fat. It's easier to avoid them altogether sometimes instead of trying to fit them into your calorie limits.

Drinking water is extremely important for losing fat. Your body needs a way to get rid of any fat that you're losing, and it does this primarily through having water carry it out through your digestive system.

If you're not drinking water and using the restroom regularly, you won't be losing that belly fat as easily. Really, you can try just about any diet if you want to go with a premade one, but the most important thing is that you focus on getting in more protein and fewer carbs. Carbs are what's causing the excess buildup of fat in your belly, which is why you can't see your abs. Cutting back on that may be all you really need.

Avoid Foods That Bloat Your Belly

Sometimes, even if you have visible abs, you might notice that you can't see them. This is usually the result of eating bloating foods that can cause your stomach region to look larger than it normally is.

You should try your best to avoid these foods because not only do they cause you to bloat up, but they can also put more gas in your intestinal system, which can cause discomfort.

Naturally, one of the most common bloating drinks is anything carbonated. This could be sodas, beers, sparkling water, anything that has some fizz to it. These drinks contain gas which your body has to put through its digestive system, which will cause bloating pretty quickly.

They're also simply not healthy for you, so you could probably stand to avoid drinking them anyway. Next, you should try to cut back on beans. Beans are fairly healthy for you, so it's not necessarily bad to eat them, but they do cause bloating.

When your body digests them, it releases gas that can cause cramping and definitely causes bloating. Cutting back on these will have you looking more defined on a regular basis, potentially revealing some abs.

Some people don't realize it, but you might actually be lactose intolerant without knowing it. It varies in severity, so you might not have horrible reactions to dairy products, but you can still get an upset stomach from them.

Lactose intolerance basically means that your body can't quite process lactose, a major component of dairy, adequately enough, which causes bloating, stomach cramps, and more.

Try switching to some milk alternatives and dairy free products if this might be an issue for you. Many adults enjoy some alcoholic beverages every now and then, but be warned, alcoholic drinks will often bloat you.

Most cocktails and light drinks like beer and wine are mixed with things like carbonated beverages or sweet syrups that will make you bloat up pretty bad. Alcohol can also make you develop a bit of a gut, which could hide your abs for a longer period of time.

By cutting out these foods and drinks, not only will you save yourself from uncomfortable and unflattering bloating, but you'll also prevent yourself from gaining weight, since most of these are unhealthy anyways. Eating clean is so important for having those six pack abs, so as long as you're sticking to a good diet, you're going to be fine.

Fitness Game Plan - 2020

Be Consistent to Carve Out Your Six Pack Abs

When you have a goal that you're really striving towards, it can be a relief once you finally reach it. Six pack abs are a common goal for many people's fitness ideals, and once they reach it, some people get a little too comfortable.

They go back to their old diets and stop exercising as much, only to find that one day they're gone again. In order to really achieve that six pack look, you need to be consistent.

One aspect of consistency is not getting complacent when you reach your goal. It seems like many people think that once they reach that point, they're going to lock it in there and it won't really require maintenance.

In reality, it does require upkeep and you have to keep on working out to maintain it. Chances are, by the time you get to the point of having abs, you're going to enjoy working out a lot more than you did when you started, so it shouldn't be too hard to keep it going.

Consistency isn't just a factor when you reach your goals, though. It's also crucial when you're on the path to your goals. It's a very common thing for people to give up on diets or workout programs because they're not seeing the results they want fast enough.

They think that after a month of working out they're going to have a six pack, while when they started, they had a beer gut. This is simply an unrealistic expectation. It takes time and consistency to make serious changes like that.

It might take months, it might take over a year, but once you reach that point, all you have to do is maintain. You can't just go back to drinking sodas every day and eating junk food all the time just because you felt like you weren't getting results fast enough.

It just doesn't work that way. By staying on top of your diet and exercise, staying away from cheat days, and not skipping workouts, you're going to see massive changes in your physical fitness.

You're undertaking a substantial project by getting into great shape, but that's fine. Fitness isn't a race - it's a marathon. If you have the right diet and you're going to the gym, you're going to see the results you want like six pack abs as long as you keep up with it and don't falter.

Regardless of how you get your six pack (or even eight-pack) set of abs, it will take a bit of time to see the results, depending on where you're starting from in your fitness journey.

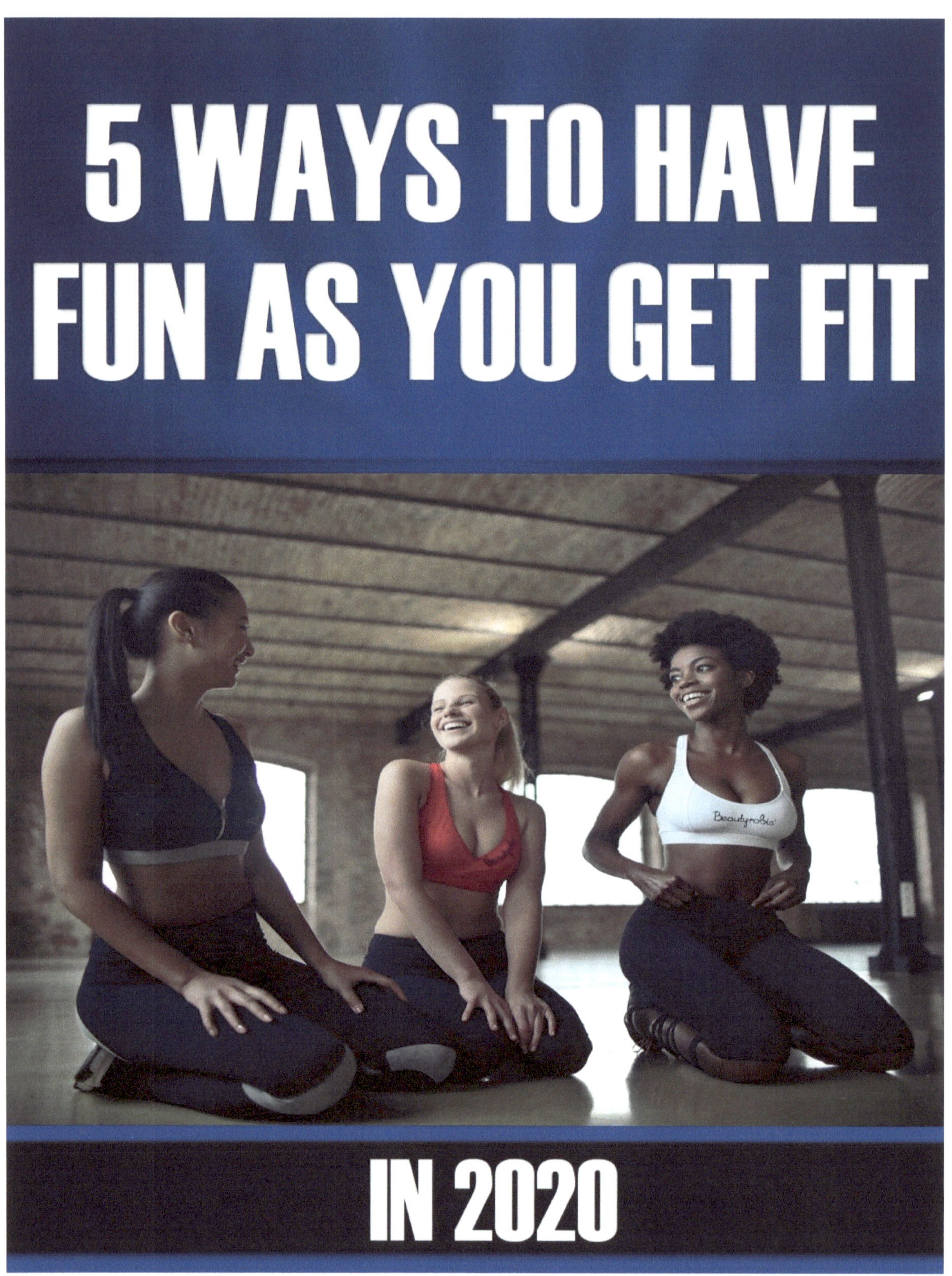
5 WAYS TO HAVE
FUN AS YOU GET FIT
IN 2020

5 Ways to Have Fun as You Get Fit In 2020

There are some things we do because we want to live our best lives. Getting fit is one of them. It isn't necessarily a fun thing to do if you just force yourself to eat right and do boring exercises every day.

If you don't approach it from a place of enthusiasm, it will be very hard for you to maintain any sort of consistency over the course of weeks, months, and years. Instead, you'll begin to dread doing it and you'll procrastinate and avoid it whenever possible.

Walk in Interesting Destinations

Walking on a treadmill in a gym is unbearably boring. Nobody likes getting in shape by walking the same speed on a flat surface staring blankly at the wall, at best with music coming in through headphones.

It makes things tedious, and when you have to do something tedious, more often than not you're going to stop doing it. If you really want to commit to fitness and not be bored to death while doing it, get outside and walk in some interesting places instead.

There are so many good places to walk all around the world. No matter where you live, you're bound to have some place good not too far away and have fun while you get fit. One common place is the park.

Almost every city or town has a park that you can go visit, and they often have dedicated paths and trails just for people who want to run or walk around. You can park and go through that whole path and it might end up being over a mile before you even realize it.

Some cities have botanical gardens open to the public, and this is a great option, too. They're essentially much nicer parks, full of flowers and beautiful trees. Having this scenery makes the long walk so much more bearable because you're actually seeing things that you like, and as the seasons progress, you'll be able to see all the flora changing.

One of the best options is hiking. If you're fortunate enough to live near a nature reserve or natural park with hiking trails, it's highly recommended to hike through there. It has changing slopes and elevations, so you're going to get better cardio than you would on a treadmill anyway, but it also has the added bonus of better sights and a feeling of accomplishment.

If you're going to go hiking or even going through some park trails, be sure to know what kind of animals live in that area. Whether it be insects, snakes, or mammals, there could be some dangerous life out there, and you'll want to be sure to steer clear of it no matter what.

Fitness Game Plan - 2020

Your best bet is to not touch any plants or animals that you see out in nature, because you have no idea what they're like, what they can do, and if they have any diseases. Try bringing a friend along for added company and added protection and bring along a camera so you can have fun snapping pictures along the way!

Get Lost in an Audiobook or Video Series as You Work Out

Whether you walk outside or inside on a treadmill, there are things that you can do to help pass the time as you walk. In recent years, tons of forms of media have become accessible at the touch of a button with smart phones, and that media makes working out a breeze, where you hardly even notice half an hour passing by.

One of the best examples of this is audiobooks. Amazon has one of the largest audiobook services, Audible, which has a massive library of audiobooks. If you're not familiar, it's an audio file of a professional voice actor or celebrity reading a book out loud in full, so you can read a book without having to really look at it.

This has helped people on long drives and flights, but it's also great at the gym. For avid readers, this helps you fit working out into your day without having to sacrifice time you would've rather spent delving into a book.

For more popular texts, some of the voice actors that they bring in to read them are incredible, and make it more immersive. All the while, you can be hiking or riding an exercise bike at the gym.

Various video series are also easily accessible these days. Things like Netflix, Hulu, and Disney+ have given people the ability to watch almost all their favorite shows straight from their phone with their apps.

Combining this with a treadmill at the gym is a fantastic way to get in shape. If you can get your hands on some Bluetooth headphones that work with your phone, you can get your phone to play your favorite show or movie, have the audio come through your wireless headphones so you don't have to worry about the wire, and prop up your phone on the treadmill while you walk.

You can binge watch whatever you'd like and before you know it, you've spent the last hour walking on the treadmill. It's important that you make your workouts enjoyable so that you'll stay committed to doing them.

If it's boring and hard, that doesn't mean it's going to work - it just means you're inevitably going to get tired of it. Some people enjoy just running, but not all people do. Using little tricks like watching a show or listening to a book might be what you need to keep on pushing through those boring walks at the gym.

Fitness Game Plan - 2020

Use Your Pet's Needs to Help You Get Fit

Any dog owner knows that they need a lot of attention, and larger breeds definitely need their walks. Sitting around cooped up inside all day isn't good for them, but it isn't good for you either.

If you sit around all day, you and your dog are going to get overweight and out of shape, so you need to go on some walks together in order to stay fit. Walking your dog is one of the best ways to bond with them.

They'll get super excited at the mere mention of a "walk" and you'll get some exercise in yourself. Take them around the park, up and down a residential street, whatever you prefer.

As long as you're both getting cardio in, that's great. Make sure whenever you go on walks to bring any necessary bags or other items for when your dog uses the restroom, though, so you don't end up leaving waste behind in public spaces.

Even if you don't have your own dog, you might be able to help one of your friends by walking theirs. If they work a lot or don't like taking them, you can do so to help your friend, spend time with their dog, and get in shape.

For all parties, it's a positive outcome. Something you also might consider is volunteering to help walk shelter dogs. They're often cooped up in their cages day in and day out, and they don't get all the attention they need due to the low staff numbers.

By volunteering, you could really be helping them out more than you know. You can walk a bunch of different dogs all in the same day, giving them exercise, socialization, and a chance to play around.

You'll get a sense of satisfaction knowing you got to help and make a difference, but you'll also get some much needed cardio from either running with them or holding them from going too fast and from walking long distances.

No matter what you choose to do, you're guaranteed to lose some weight from doing dog walking. If you get really good at it, you could consider charging people to do it on the side to pull in some extra cash while you get fit.

Managing multiple dogs at the same time can be stressful, but all that pulling will certainly work out your arms and leave you feeling sore the next day.

Find an Exercise Buddy to Partner Up with You

Going to the gym, especially as a beginner, can be stressful when you're on your own. You walk in, you see people in better shape than you lifting heavy weights, and you don't even know where to start.

Fitness Game Plan - 2020

You can feel lost. There are often cliques of people that know each other from going there for a long time, and you almost feel like you're being watched as the new member. In order to make things much, much easier (and more fun), bring a friend to the gym to be your dedicated exercise partner.

Being the only new person walking in can make you feel like you stick out like a sore thumb, but with someone else by your side, especially someone that you're friends with, all of that fear goes away and you feel much more comfortable.

One of the best things about having a gym partner is that you can hold each other accountable. When you don't want to go to the gym, there's no pressure not to if you're the only one that goes at that time.

However, if you have a friend that can text you and call you who you know is going to be meeting you there, you have to pull it together and go to the gym anyway. Keeping on track is extremely important for fitness.

It helps a lot if your gym partner is experienced in working out. They can then act almost like your personal trainer, sharing their knowledge with you and helping you correct your form or certain workouts, helping you ensure that what you're doing is going to see results.

Many beginners are too nervous to ask for help and end up doing exercises wrong in such a way that they're not really going to make progress with them. They can also supply you with good workout routines to follow if you don't have one already.

Most of all, a gym partner can make the experience fun. Even in the bad times when you're sore and uncomfortable and want to give up, you can crack a joke with them and at least put a smile on your face instead of just angrily packing up and leaving.

In the good times, you're sharing new personal records with each other and lifting each other up to keep on improving. This will keep you motivated to keep working out and keep you coming back to the gym time after time.

Make a Game Out of It

Fitness is often boring if you don't find it inherently fun. Some people really like running or weightlifting on their own, and don't mind just going with some music and working out.

Others need a bit more motivation than that, so to keep yourself interested in getting in shape, you should make a game out of it to make things more fun. There are lots of things that you can do, primarily from apps, to help get you in shape.

One of the most popular apps that got people walking around was Pokémon GO. It encouraged users to walk around in order to find and catch Pokémon, as well as come across various stops, usually points of interest in a city, in order to gain items.

Fitness Game Plan - 2020

You can also walk to hatch eggs that will hatch after either 2 km, 5 km, or 10 km. This game alone is a great way to get you walking. If you live in a city, you can find Facebook groups for the game in your specific city, who will post updates about Pokémon that are popping up in the area.

You can plan out a route that you can walk around the cities to hit up different stops and even battle at gyms along the way. There are other games that people love to play for fitness, as well.

For example, geocaching still has a rather large active community of players that are still hiding and finding caches to this day. If you're not familiar with it, geocaching is a game people play in which you use GPS coordinates to find hidden caches, usually containing a logbook and some trinkets.

You can sign off your name in it can leave it there for the next lucky person to find. This is a great game for fitness because it involves a lot of hiking, which is great for cardio. It also allows you to get a sense of adventure, like you're searching for treasure.

These caches are located all around the world, so you're sure to have some in your area. You can sign up on their website and use apps to find the cache locations. Some people have found success in fitness based video games.

In these, they have you perform various cardio-intensive actions in order to complete objectives and advance through the story. This is a better option for those that prefer to stay inside, but still want to get a fun workout in.

Remember, getting fit doesn't have to be boring. You can practice fitness routines while having a lot of fun and getting your body in shape. Think of it as a dual physical and emotional well-being process.

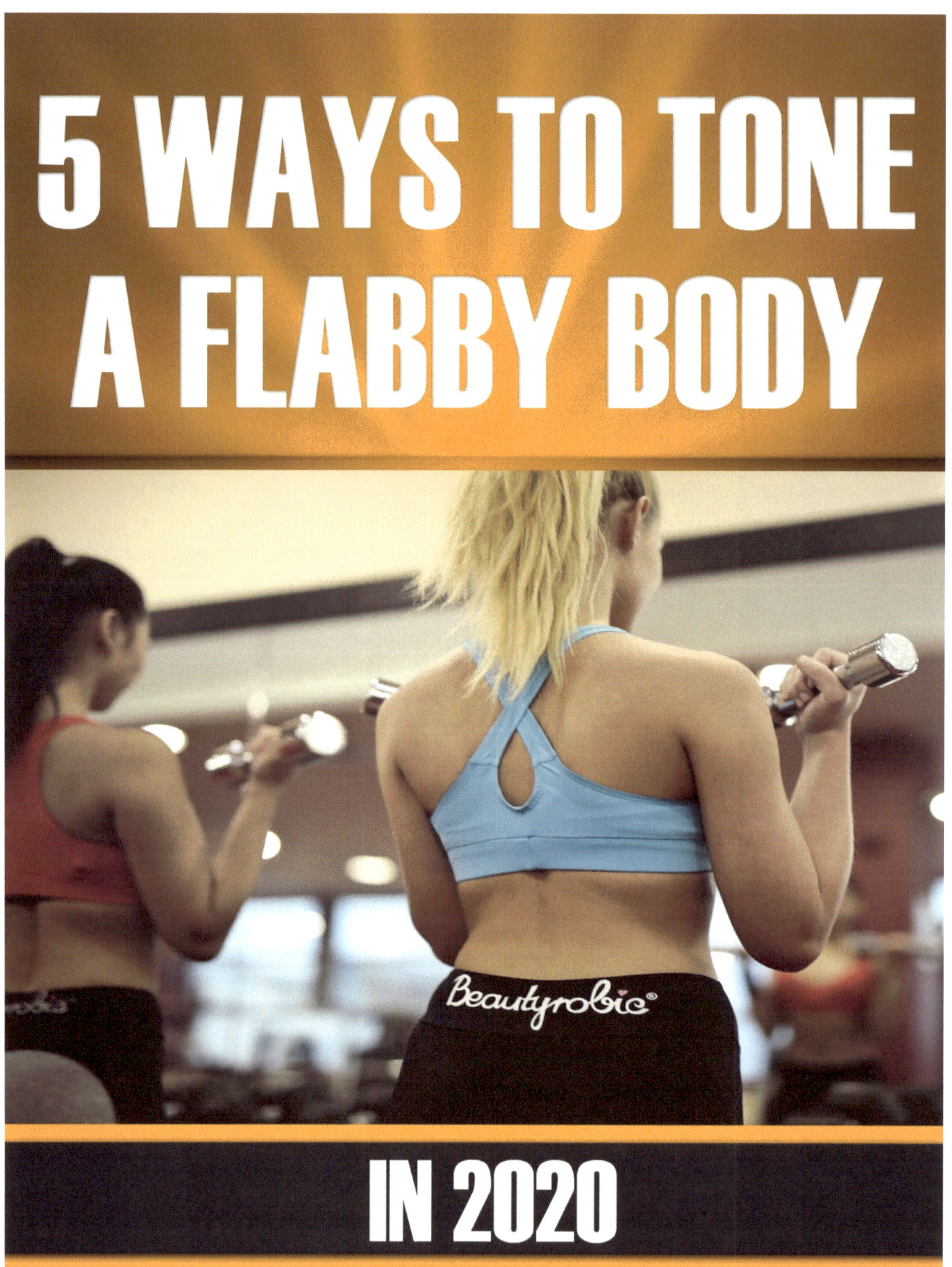
5 WAYS TO TONE
A FLABBY BODY
IN 2020

5 Ways to Tone a Flabby Body in 2020

While there's no proven way to spot train one area for fat burning, it's very possible to spot train one specific muscle group for toning. So as long as you're being consistent with an all over body fat burning regimen, your efforts to tone up certain parts of your body with targeted exercises should pay off.

There are many trouble spots people usually want to focus on when toning up. Toning up doesn't mean the same as bulking, so you don't have to worry about growth if you don't want to. It's more about the shape and firmness of the muscle, not its size.

How to Tone Your Arms

Arms can be a source of shame for many people. Depending on how fat is distributed throughout your body, you may or may not have a bit of extra skin and fat around your arms, often around the tricep or underarm area.

Arms can be a particularly hard part of the body to tone up, since it's not just dependent on losing weight like it is with belly fat. Instead, you need to focus on lifting weights in order to tone up your arms.

Triceps are the most common problem area for people's arms. You might have noticed a bit of extra skin hanging down from your arms if you hold them out to the side, called batwings, and that's just a lack of definition in your tricep.

By putting on more muscle in that area, you'll be able to firm it up and reduce the amount of loose skin. People often worry about looking too muscular, but rest assured, that won't be the case.

It just takes a bit of healthy muscle to look toned. There are plenty of tricep workouts to do in order to tone this area, with one of the most common ones being dips. Dips can be done just about anywhere with various levels of difficulty depending on how strong you are.

They can be done by holding onto a slightly elevated surface behind you, with your feet out in front of you on the ground. You let your body come down, and then push yourself back up.

This should give you a pretty good burning feeling in your triceps. For those who are a bit more fitness inclined, there are more advanced and difficult forms of tricep dips that you can do.

Some will support their whole bodyweight on two bars and dip their body down that way, while some will even add on weight and do this for added difficulty. Either way, this is a surefire way to tone up your arms.

Fitness Game Plan - 2020

One often overlooked part of your arms is your forearms. People are always focused on their biceps or their underarms, and they forget that there's a pretty significant amount of arm muscles below the elbow.

By doing simple things like grip strength testers, you can tone up your forearms and give your overall arms a bit of a nicer look, though some people just won't be able to tell exactly what you did.

Plus, the muscle strength will support you and help prevent injuries such as tennis elbow whenever you have strength in your arms that can support everyday activities. You may not even think about this until it becomes a problem and you're forced to work that area out as a form of recovery and repair.

How to Tone Your Legs

Many people store a bit of their extra fat in their legs. Often times, this can be seen in the quadriceps or hamstrings, but also a bit in the hips. Now, having fat on your legs isn't necessarily unhealthy, but excess fat certainly is.

This can make things like moving around more difficult, and getting into some kinds of clothes, like jeans, a bit of a tight fit. In order to avoid those kinds of problems, you need to tone up your legs.

There are plenty of ways to do this, and you don't necessarily have to do all of them or just one of them - you can mix and match these as you'd like. The first and most common way to tone up legs is by dieting.

If your body stores fat mostly in the legs, then dieting will surely help your leg mass go down. Cutting back on your overall calorie intake as well as managing your macromolecules will help you lose weight and will shed a good amount of the fat in your legs.

Of course, cardio is also a great option. Cardio is incredibly versatile, so you should be able to find something that you like doing in order to help you tone up your legs. Naturally, when people think of cardio, they tend to think about cardio machines like treadmills or exercise bikes.

These are fine options, but they're not your only options. There are plenty of other leg-driven cardio routines out there that you might find more enjoyable. Biking, for example, uses a lot of leg energy and is great for getting your legs toned.

Biking short distances instead of driving can help you tone up and save money on things like gas, so it can be a great option if you live in a more suburban or urban area. Other than that, things like hiking or playing recreational sports are sure to get your blood pumping, your legs moving, and your lower body more toned.

Fitness Game Plan - 2020

They're also just great ways to get connected with new people and enjoy a new hobby. Making cardio enjoyable is by far the best way of getting in shape, because having fun with new friends will always be better than jogging on a treadmill for a few hours.

Finally, there are always simple forms of weightlifting. You don't necessarily need to use weights for leg training, especially if you're looking to tone up rather than put on muscle. Doing high reps of bodyweight squats is a simple and easy way to get your legs toned up fast.

How to Tone Your Stomach

The stomach is by far the most common problem area for excess fat. People are constantly worried about having a "gut" or "belly," and want to tone it down as quickly as possible.

Often times, people look for a flat stomach or [even abs](#) as the number one sign of fitness, so it's certainly an important thing to tone up. From a more health-based perspective, belly fat is one of the most dangerous kinds, being more of an indicator for things like heart problems than any other kind of fat.

The most useful solution for belly fat is simple weight loss through dieting. It's common for people to believe that exercise is what gets you in shape, but that's not necessarily the case.

Exercise does help, but abs are made (or covered up) in the kitchen. The calories you burn with an intense workout can be undone by a single soda or dessert. Instead of focusing on exercising as hard as possible and then rewarding yourself with unhealthy food, simply eat less unhealthy food.

Getting rid of things like liquid calories from sweet drinks or eating multiple servings of desserts can help you shed pounds so quickly. If you want the real fast track to getting rid of belly fat, dieting is your best option.

When combined with dieting, exercise is also a great helper in getting your stomach toned. When you're using one specific body part a lot, it'll burn fat around that area the most.

There are plenty of exercises out there that you can do to help your stomach fat disappear. Abdominal exercises are going to be your best bet here. Usually when people think of this they default to something like sit-ups, which aren't really that fun, and in fact, aren't really the best ab exercise.

There are tons of more enjoyable ab exercises that will still get you in shape without feeling like you're in gym class again. Get together with a buddy and do crunches with a medicine ball tossed after each rep.

Fitness Game Plan - 2020

Lay with your feet touching and when you're at the top, toss the medicine ball to your partner. Wait until they're back up after their rep, catch it, and repeat. Tossing around a heavy ball tends to make things a bit more enjoyable, as does doing something with a friend. Another great ab exercise is yoga, which provides you with less stress about working out harder, and more relaxation and meditation.

How to Tone Your Back

The back, for both men and women, is a great muscle to tone up. A toned, muscular back is what absolutely completes any summer body type look, separating you from some people who just hit the gym every now and then.

Toning up your back can help you get rid of things like love handles, as well as give you a bit more of a "V" shaped body that makes you look much better. For the most part, people tend to not store a lot of fat in their backs.

It mostly ends up being a lack of muscle that makes it look untoned. So, for the most part, toning up your back involves a good amount of weightlifting in order to get it looking strong.

There are tons of different exercises that you'll want to do or try in order to get your back toned up. If you can do them, pullups are always a great back exercise. They put a lot of work into your lats, which are the upper side parts of your back that give you that "V" shape.

Pullups can be done even at home with a cheap piece of equipment that attaches to your door frame, so you don't even need a gym membership for those. If you can't do pullups properly, lots of gyms have an assisted pullup machine, in which you can adjust the amount of weight that it helps push you with to make the pullups easier.

Rows are a big part of back toning. Whether it be a common low row machine, or bent over rows with a barbell, rowing is great for your lower and middle back. This basically covers the muscles that aren't the lats, but are still important for having your back look toned.

Rowing is a very simple motion, in that all you're really doing is pulling something towards your stomach, so that your back does the work. Rows can be a bit dangerous if you don't do them properly, though.

Pulling with your back should be done with an appropriate amount of weight and should be done in a controlled way. If you're flinging the weight towards yourself as hard as possible, you're probably going to injure yourself long before you put on any muscle.

There are tons of variations of these two common workouts that make back exercises very versatile. From lateral pulldowns to replace pullups to all kinds of dumbbell exercises to replace rows, you're sure to find something that you'll enjoy.

Fitness Game Plan - 2020

How to Tone Your Buttocks

Plenty of people store a bit of excess fat in their glutes. While having fat there is usually pretty normal, you can tell when it's a bit too much. Having some muscle behind that fat can make your glutes more firm, and it also helps a lot with day to day life in terms of mobility.

There are plenty of ways to tone up your buttocks with simple bodyweight exercises and minor weightlifting. One fun way to tone up your glutes is through swimming. Swimming is a surprisingly good form of cardio, as long as you're actually doing it for exercise.

By swimming laps instead of just floating around for awhile, you're actually doing a lot of cardio. It's pretty low-impact work so you don't feel as sore, but you do get the benefits. Swimming combines using your glutes as you swim with fat-burning cardio in order to give you a lot more definition.

Of course, there are plenty of [bodyweight exercises](#) that you can do at home as well. Squats are by far the most important bodyweight exercises for toned glutes. If done with proper form, you should feel it distinctly in your glutes when you drive up from the ground, and doing this for high amounts of reps will have you feeling sore in no time.

You can also add difficulty by holding a medicine ball or even doing weighted squats with a barbell and all. Another exercise that's great for your glutes is lunges. Lunges alone are great for your legs as a whole, and by doing twist lunges you can even get an ab workout in.

However, for your glutes, they're fantastic. They're a bit lighter on your knees, and you're actually moving while you do them, so it feels less static and boring. You can hold dumbbells on either side of you while you do these for added intensity.

You can't go wrong with gym machines. When you walk around the machines at your gym, you'll find that they'll almost always have stickers on them telling you what body part this machine helps with, and how exactly to do the exercise.

Pay attention to these so that you save yourself from sitting there for minutes on end figuring out what body parts go where. Find yourself a nice glute machine at your gym and get to work. Chances are, it has one or two that you'll find enjoyable enough.

Make sure you're implementing a toning strategy for all of the important areas of your body. You don't to have only a few helping support your frame. You want to give each muscle the ability to lend help whenever you need it.

Final Thoughts

Patience is a highly underrated virtue… and it's of paramount importance when it comes to transforming your body and reclaiming your health. Christian author, Joyce Meyer once said, "Patience is not the ability to wait, but the ability to keep a good attitude while waiting."

There is immense wisdom in this quote and it's something that every single person should remember when striving for a worthy goal. It's especially more important to those who are trying to lose weight and get fit.

Why you need patience

Flip open any fitness magazine and all you'll ever see are articles about what diets to adopt or what exercises you should incorporate in your training regimen. It's mostly technical info to help you achieve your goal… but very often, these publications neglect the mental aspect of fitness and body transformation.

If you're trying to lose weight, it will take time. The average person can only lose about 2 pounds of fat a week. If you're 30 pounds overweight, that will amount to about 15 weeks, which is almost 4 months.

So many enthusiastic folks make a New Year's resolution to lose weight and they believe that it'll be over and done with by end-January. They don't even realize that it may take them until the end of April (or longer) to achieve their goal.

In the event their weight loss progress plateaus (very common when losing weight), it will take even longer to get to their ideal weight. The goal might only materialize in June. That's half the year gone!

Do you have the patience to wait so long?

This is a very important question to ask yourself.

What happens if you lack patience?

For starters, you'll feel like a failure. You'll feel unworthy because your efforts yield no fruit. Working out is tiring. Sticking to a clean diet requires self-discipline. It's a lot of effort.

Fitness Game Plan - 2020

When you don't see fast results despite your best efforts, you may feel like what you're doing is useless and you're destined to be fat. This is where most people throw in the towel and believe that the goal is beyond their reach.

They blame their big bones, their laziness, their genetics, etc. Nothing could be further from the truth.

They just lack patience. With time they'll achieve their goals if they stay on track.

Tracking your progress

It's a very good habit to keep a journal to track your fitness journey. Be as detailed as possible and write down what you eat, your weight, bodyfat percentage, your workout sessions, etc.

The goal is to make continuous improvements daily. You should be pushing yourself to keep beating your personal bests. Clean up your diet to the best of your ability. Give it your all in your workouts. Be as compliant to your fitness plan as possible.

You must find joy in the small improvements. Over time, all these will add up to a massive difference. Take photos of your body once every two weeks. These photos will be proof that your body is slowly transforming.

See them daily and motivate yourself to keep going. If you hate starting over, then don't stop. Harness the power of patience and dogged determination to stay on track even when your goal is nothing but a mirage on the horizon.

You'll ultimately get there, if you have patience. Your patience will achieve more than your force. Keep going. You can do this and achieve your fitness goal in 2020!

Fitness Game Plan - 2020

Recommended Resources

Throughout this book, you have seen words highlighted and may wonder what that is. Those words match the words here and each word is followed by a link to an additional resource that you may find useful. Some are products to enhance your training; others are books on a topic to provide you with more information on that topic if you are interested in learning more about it.

Bodyweight exercises - https://www.amazon.com/gp/product/B07YZQRMN6

Stable Bar - https://amzn.to/36N6adQ

HIIT Training - https://www.amazon.com/gp/product/B06XVFDKV9

Crossfit - https://www.amazon.com/gp/product/B01FELQFKS

Meditation - https://www.amazon.com/gp/product/B07NC974SF

Yoga - https://www.amazon.com/gp/product/B07H5G2PJH

Learn How - https://www.amazon.com/gp/product/B06Y4BQDJN

Strength Training - https://www.amazon.com/gp/product/B01MRDBASE

Toning Up - https://www.amazon.com/gp/product/B075QXXYM8

Bulking Up - https://www.amazon.com/gp/product/1539352226

Protein - https://www.amazon.com/gp/product/B073G9DDDF

Protein - https://www.amazon.com/gp/product/1540731227

Injuries - https://www.amazon.com/gp/product/B06Y4BQDJN

Cardio - https://www.amazon.com/gp/product/B00PD8B6ES

High Intensity - https://www.amazon.com/gp/product/B06XVFDKV9

Daily Routine - https://www.amazon.com/gp/product/B07PPKFFDP

Proper Sleep - https://www.amazon.com/gp/product/B07ZBKHSF9

Proper Amounts of Sleep - https://www.amazon.com/gp/product/B07K2CVLSL

Burn the Fat - https://www.amazon.com/gp/product/B07MHLGPC8

Lose Weight - https://www.amazon.com/gp/product/B07SFWVGTY

Heart Health - https://www.amazon.com/gp/product/B00WRCHCRS

Lower Carb Diet - https://www.amazon.com/gp/product/B07X9HDWR6

Strength Training - https://www.amazon.com/gp/product/B075QXXYM8

Fitness Game Plan - 2020

Gut Health - https://www.amazon.com/gp/product/B072272RVD

Gut Bacteria - https://www.amazon.com/gp/product/1537314823

Weight and Fat Gain - https://www.amazon.com/gp/product/B081XKDZNJ

Cut Back - https://www.amazon.com/gp/product/B07YBKJ586

Cut Out Any and All Sweet and Sugary Drinks - https://www.amazon.com/gp/product/1536868981

Fat Burning - https://www.amazon.com/gp/product/B06XQH9KCV

Home Gym - https://www.amazon.com/gp/product/1539711234

Exercising Naturally - https://www.amazon.com/gp/product/153550000X

Don't Require You To Use Weights - https://www.amazon.com/gp/product/B07YZQRMN6

Healthier Options - https://www.amazon.com/gp/product/1720209774

Abs - https://www.amazon.com/Get-Ripped-Abs-Best-Six-Pack-ebook/dp/B00M2CYANW

Planks - https://www.amazon.com/gp/product/B06Y1561YQ

Belly Fat - https://www.amazon.com/Basics-Blasting-Belly-Fat-Benefits/dp/1539550079

Cutting Sugary - https://www.amazon.com/gp/product/B074D4WL2T

Healthier Option - https://www.amazon.com/gp/product/1720209774

Dairy Free Products - https://www.amazon.com/gp/product/B076N1Z3MW

Walk - https://www.amazon.com/gp/product/B078G424FB

Walk - https://www.amazon.com/gp/product/B00S4ALBMO

Dedicated Exercise Partner - https://www.amazon.com/gp/product/B06Y3FYXWC

Fitness - https://www.amazon.com/gp/product/B06XQH9KCV

Fat Burning - https://www.amazon.com/gp/product/B06XQH9KCV

Lifting Weights - https://www.amazon.com/gp/product/B075QXXYM8

Grip Strength Testers - https://amzn.to/2M69LLV

Lose Weight - https://www.amazon.com/gp/product/B06XQH9KCV

Even Abs - https://www.amazon.com/gp/product/B00XLOL52E

Toned Muscular Back - https://www.amazon.com/gp/product/1539352226

Weightlifting - https://www.amazon.com/gp/product/1539534545

Fitness Game Plan - 2020

Bodyweight Exercises - https://www.amazon.com/Functional-Fitness-Explained-Everyday-Easier-ebook/dp/B07FK5Q77R

About the Author

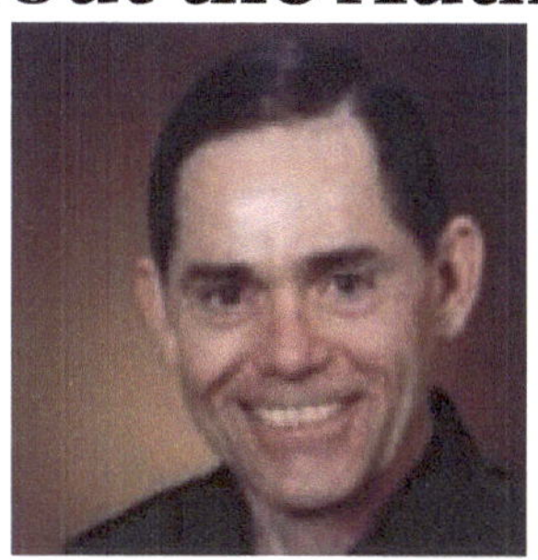

I have published numerous books on Amazon (both for Kindle and in paperback), along with other publishing platforms.

While most of my books are on health and fitness in general, I also write on baby boomer and older citizen health issues and have a recent interest in creating and printing journals/ planners and other printable products.

Besides my own writing, I also ghostwrite ebooks, books, reports, articles, blogs and do Kindle conversions for clients on a variety of topics.

Go to my website at http://ronknesswriting.com for more information or to submit a quote. For a complete list of my books, go to https://www.amazon.com/Ron-Kness/e/B0072M6PYO.

Today my wife and I are retired from our careers and live in Queen Creek, AZ. I now write as a retirement business where you'll find me happily sitting in my office typing away on my laptop as I work on my next book or ghostwriting project . . . that is if we are not traveling on a cruise ship - our new-found mode of travel.